Let's Do Lunch

*Eating All the Calories and Carbs
You Want to Lose Weight!*

ROGER TROY WILSON

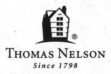

THOMAS NELSON
Since 1798

NASHVILLE DALLAS MEXICO CITY RIO DE JANEIRO BEIJING

Published in Nashville, Tennessee, by Thomas Nelson. Thomas Nelson is a registered trademark of Thomas Nelson, Inc.

This book was previously published as *Let's Do Lunch*. Copyright © 2003, 2005 by Sunshine Publications, Inc. It has been revised and updated.

Let's Do Lunch™ is a licensed trademark. It is owned entirely by Sunshine Publications, Inc.

Thomas Nelson, Inc. titles may be purchased in bulk for educational, business, fund-raising, or sales promotional use. For information, please e-mail SpecialMarkets@ThomasNelson.com.

ISBN 978-0-7852-2939-1 (Revised and Updated Edition)

Library of Congress Cataloging-in-Publication

Wilson, Roger Troy.
    Let's do lunch : you'll never have to diet again / Roger Troy Wilson.
      p. cm.
    ISBN: 0-7852-1321-X
  1. Reducing diets. 2. Luncheons. I. Title.
    RM222.2.W462 2005
    613.2'5—dc22

                2005012265

Printed in the United States of America

09 10 11 12 13 QW 9 8 7 6 5 4 3 2

This book is dedicated to my brother, Steven Neil Wilson, who died August 15, 1992, after suffering from terrible stomach cancer. His death, however, was anything but painful. He sat up in bed, opened his eyes, got the biggest smile on his face I had ever seen, opened his arms as wide as they would go . . . and at that very moment he died—with the smile still on his face. He loved Jesus with all of his heart and had been rebaptized in the Pacific Ocean just before his death.

I want everyone who reads this book to know how very much I loved my brother and how proud I am to have shared his life with him. I believe he will be with me forever. His memory guides my endeavors to help God save the lives of people all over the world who are losing their battle with obesity, as well as to help our heavenly Father with those who want to lose a few pounds so that they live healthier and happier lives.

In my brother's name, I am pledging 100 percent of my profits from this book to churches, charities, and ministries to help spread God's Word throughout the world. I am making this pledge because I think it is important that I not take a profit on a blessing that God meant for everyone.

I also want to thank my wife, Anita, for her support, love, care, and concern during all of my four-hundred-pound fat years. The same kind of thanks are due my mother and father, Ruth and Orville; my children, Tyra and Ty; my grandchildren, Brandon, Dustin, and Brittany; and all the rest of my family, my wife's family, and our friends, especially Bob Lichtinger.

My wife tells me she used to worry constantly about me dying and about being alone in her older years. I'm glad she no longer needs to worry that I will die from obesity. I now know that my family and friends were embarrassed at times because of my weight, yet none of them ever let on about their uneasiness. For that, I will be forever grateful.

Roger Troy Wilson

Contents

Before You Start
this Program

Words of Caution

Consult Your Physician Before Starting the
***Let's Do Lunch* Eating Program.**

Before starting this, or any other diet program, you should schedule an appointment with your physician for a full consultation, exam, and approval. If you are currently taking medication or are ill, it is imperative that your physician approves your participation in this program. This program is not to be construed as any form of diagnosis, prescription, or treatment. If you do not choose to see your physician, neither the author nor Sunshine Publications, Inc., nor the publisher, nor any other person or entity disseminating or selling this material can assume any responsibility whatsoever for your actions or omissions.

The publisher and author do not directly or indirectly dispense medical advice or prescribe the use of diet as a form of treatment for sickness without medical approval. Nutritionists and other experts in the fields of health and nutrition hold widely varying views. It is not the intent of the publisher or author to diagnose or prescribe. The intent is only to offer information to help you cooperate with your doctor in your mutual quest for health. In the event you use this information without your doctor's approval, you are prescribing for yourself, which is your constitutional right, but the publisher and author assume no responsibility. Also, because there may be some individual risk involved, the publisher and author are not responsible for any adverse effects or consequences resulting from the use or misuse of any of the requirements, suggestions, preparations, procedures, recipes, or other content in this book.

Personal Experience and Verified Results

The author is stating in this book what happened to him, his wife, his mother, and his agent, as well as what he believes. His physicians are Dr. Neil Hoffman of Minneapolis, Minnesota, and Dr. Eli Farri of Fort Myers, Florida. Both witnessed his weight loss.

Testimonials from Others

Throughout this book you will find testimonial statements from other people who have used the *Let's Do Lunch* program with great success. These are real statements from real people. Permission has been granted to use these statements; only their initials and state names are used to help ensure personal privacy.

Recommendations

The names of foods, menus, and restaurants identified in this program were specially selected by the author, who found them to be the tastiest and healthiest foods for inclusion in his *Let's Do Lunch* eating plan. None of the brands, menus, or restaurants have been paid a promotional consideration to be included in *Let's Do Lunch*, nor does their inclusion constitute an endorsement, recommendation, or other suggestion by them as to any aspect of *Let's Do Lunch*. All such products and company names are trademarks or registered trademarks of their respective holders.

A Comment About Exercising

You can lose weight with the *Let's Do Lunch* program without exercising—or you can lose it even faster by engaging in some physical activity. In any case, the author honestly believes that exercise is beneficial to your health. Try mixing up different activities on different days instead of just one that you do repeatedly. Just like eating only certain foods that you get sick of after time, the same exercise plan over and over can become boring. Again, please consult your physician to get his or her approval of the activity or exercise in which you intend to participate.

Trust the Plan

Do *not* portion control. I'll say it again, do *not* portion control. If you do, you are destined for failure. You *must* eat until full, and *trust* that *Let's Do Lunch* will make you feel less hungry with each day that goes by . . . to the point that your body will *force* you to eat less and less, consume fewer and fewer calories, and lose all the weight you want.

Read the Book Three Times

In order to remember everything, please read chapters 2 through 6 at least three times.

Imperative to Remember!

When I was morbidly obese, for approximately thirty years, the problems I had with losing weight involved being hungry all the time as well as craving certain fattening foods.

But then, with *Let's Do Lunch*, I was never hungry because I ate until I was full, and my cravings for those certain fattening foods were totally eliminated because I was eating in all the food groups, including starchy and sweet carbs.

I thought I was home free . . . not! Why? Because even though I didn't crave those certain fattening foods, I found myself just *wanting* to eat them because I loved them. I loved eating bread, pizza, and French fries, and I loved eating chocolate, ice cream, and doughnuts.

I know you can relate to this because food is one of the most important parts of our lives! So I had to come up with a way to think about these foods whenever I became weak or just wanted to enjoy eating them again even though I didn't crave them.

Here is what I came up with. If you *loved* the taste of arsenic, and yet you didn't crave it, would you still want to eat it, knowing that it would kill you? Of course not! So why would you want to eat something you don't crave when you know it will cause you to gain weight . . . when you know it will cause you to hate the way you look and feel?

And one more thing—every *little* step you take to lose weight can become a *big* step if you continue taking those little steps. For example, if you are served a sandwich at someone's home, why eat it with two slices of bread when you get the same taste with one slice?

Every time you are ready to put something in your mouth and eat it, think about how to eat it in a less-fattening way.

When doing *Let's Do Lunch*, it is imperative to remember the above.

My sweet little Dana Hock from Detroit inspired me to write this part of the book, and I want to thank her for that inspiration.

Introduction

This Plan Is Not What You Think

It's Far Different . . . and Far Better!

When you think about losing weight, do you automatically think about being hungry? Do you think about being limited to eating only certain foods, and craving foods you should not be eating? Do you think about being deprived more than rewarded with results? If so, I have great news for you. This plan is different. You get to eat foods you love—whenever you are hungry and until you are full.

You don't have to eat foods you don't like. You are able to satisfy your cravings. You get to eat all you want of all the food groups—carbohydrates, fats, and proteins. You don't have to do things you don't like. In this plan:

- There is no exercise required.
- There are no pills to take.
- There are no carbs, calories, points, or fat grams to count.
- There are no special shakes to drink, prescribed foods or meals to eat, or portions to control.
- There are no math exercises required to convert grams to calories.
- There are no meetings to attend.

1

You start by eating until you are full. But because *Let's Do Lunch* foods stabilize your blood sugar, your body forces you to become less and less hungry with each passing day. Therefore, you begin to eat less and less, consume fewer and fewer calories, and lose weight. Also, because you are eating until full in all the food groups, *Let's Do Lunch* eliminates all of your cravings.

A plan like this is absolutely *essential* if you want to lose weight and keep it off. Any other way, and your brain will not be satisfied, and you'll be destined to just one more diet failure. I know. I've been there, done that.

My plan works. It works to help people lose weight, and it works to help people keep the weight off. Furthermore, my plan produces good health. Don't just take it from me. Take it from an expert. I've asked Ruth Davies, a dietitian and educator, to say a word to you.

An amazing story and plan for both weight loss and healthy eating awaits you. Roger Troy Wilson has spent a lifetime suffering with obesity and the related psychological and emotional devastation that accompany it. After numerous attempts with dieting utilizing liquid diets, exchange systems, high protein and low carbohydrate intakes, weekly weigh-ins, and even acupuncture, he describes himself as a "professional diet failure." Yet somehow he kept searching, and after fifteen years of experimenting with different foods, eating patterns, and eating times, he gradually began to lose weight and has managed to keep it off for many years.

His eating plan contains healthy foods in the fat, carbohydrate, and protein groups. He may well be ahead of his time and ahead of what scientists have continually sought to find as a healthy diet. He has avoided health problems such as hypertension, heart disease, and diabetes that are typically associated with obesity and continues to live a healthy, full, and satisfying life. What he has done is truly remarkable.

During my twenty-five years as a registered dietitian, counseling many individuals and groups in their dietary goals, I marvel at his accomplishment. Roger has managed to achieve a weight loss and health status that many never do. His success can be your success too. Simply follow his suggestions and ideas and incorporate them into your lifestyle. You will soon lose pounds and gain momentum from not only Roger's contagious enthusiasm and support, but from the health results that you will obtain. Wishing you the very best in your exciting and healthy journey ahead.

Ruth Davies, M.S., R.D., L.D.
Registered Dietitian
Adjunct Professor, Edison College

The Lowest Number on the Scale Is What Counts

In the business world people are always concerned about the bottom line. In the dieting world, those of us who were fat know it's really the lowest number on the scale that counts. We want *results*.

There are lots of programs out there. Some produce quick results, but not lasting ones. Some are so boring or limiting that people can't adopt them as a way of eating for longer than a few weeks. Some produce results, but with a loss of health along the way. And some place all sorts of demands and cost all sorts of investment, so that pretty soon, a person's head can be swimming in "do and don't" rules.

At the same time, we know we can't give up. Excess fat produces bad health over time. Excess fat limits us socially. It's demoralizing and discouraging. We have to stay in the fight!

We all know the statistics. Obesity rates in the United States are rising rapidly—they've gone up by 60 percent just since 1991. Diabetes, heart disease, and certain weight-related cancers are also on the rise with no foreseeable end in sight. At the same time, information about health and nutrition has exploded in recent years. Scientists are continually testing which nutrients help fight and prevent disease and how to best combine proteins, fats, and carbohydrates.

We know more about weight and dieting than ever in history. And yet we're fatter. All the knowledge in the world doesn't matter. What matters is having a program that *works*—a program that takes off the weight, keeps off the weight, and does so in a way that keeps you healthy.

That's what my plan does for me. I believe it will do the same for you.

But again, don't just take it from me. Following are three letters I received not long ago.

Dear Roger Troy:

Since reading your program, *Let's Do Lunch,* I have generated some remarkable results. Several years ago I was diagnosed as a Type 2 diabetic. Over the years I have tried many different diets without success. *Let's Do Lunch* has not only allowed me to lose 28 pounds, but I have had a remarkable drop in my glucose blood sugar readings. Since being on the *Let's Do Lunch* diet I have reduced my glucose reading by better than 20 percent.

In an attempt to control my diabetes, I always shied away from a lot of fruits and drinks like orange juice because of the sugar content. Today my diet is loaded with a variety of sweet fruits, such as grapes, and I have orange juice every morning.

The best part of this diet is I am not hungry nor am I driven by the cravings I have had on previous diets. The combination of eating all the carbs you want, along with fats and proteins, and eating until you are full is certainly unlike other diets I have tried. After you are on *Let's Do Lunch* for a few months, your body's metabolism really does change. A few weeks ago I went out for dinner to one of my favorite restaurants and had Veal Marseillaise in a very rich sauce with a side of spaghetti. In the past this had been one of my favorite meals. The intake of rich food didn't sit well with me and I did not feel good for several hours after I ate the meal. It wasn't a pleasant experience. Once you get on the *Let's Do Lunch* diet it is very difficult for you to go back and eat the way you did before.

Your book not only is a boon to dieters everywhere, but as a diabetic, I found it especially beneficial.

REGARDS,
D.J.M., TEXAS

All praise, glory, and honor to our heavenly Father and Jesus in heaven! This man not only lost weight, he gained health! Here's another encouraging word:

Dear Roger Troy:
After reading *Let's Do Lunch,* I was interested but skeptical. My fundamental problem was not being overweight, although I knew I could lose fifteen pounds to look and feel better. My real concern was my abnormally high cholesterol. For the last twenty

years, my cholesterol levels have been nearly 500. I have been counseled to use Lipitor or other antistatin drugs to lower my cholesterol. For me, this was impossible because I had a chronic condition of Hepatitis C and all the antistatin drugs created increased stress to my liver.

Nevertheless I put my "grapes in the freezer" and began the *Let's Do Lunch* program avoiding, whenever possible, high protein meals at night . . . and within two weeks I had lost ten pounds and felt much better. My clothes fit better. The more surprising results occurred after a recent blood test. My cholesterol had dropped to 268. To verify the cause and effect, I went off the diet for two weeks, gained six pounds, and my cholesterol went back up into the high 400s. I went back on the diet for three weeks and my cholesterol is once again below 300. More importantly, the good cholesterol is 134. For me, these results have been life altering and maybe life-saving.

I thank God for this gift!

SINCERELY,
S.K.H., CALIFORNIA

I was given a copy of your program about a year and a half ago and I've been following your guidelines for healthier eating ever since. I don't use the word diet—that's a bad four-letter word to us! After about 6 months on the plan, my husband had lost 35 pounds and I had lost about 15 pounds. That is my lowest weight since high school and my husband's lowest weight since college. After reaching a comfortable plateau, we have been able to maintain our loss with no appreciable effort or weight gain.

. . . Like you, we had tried many other diets through the years with no success, principally because those diets seemed to be based on rigid deprivation. *Let's Do Lunch* . . . provides alternatives and methods to curb addictive cravings. We think this is one of the fundamental concepts that makes your plan different from others and has enabled us to be successful.

The other concept that you fully understand is that it's okay to stray now and again because it's easy to get back on track and lose anything that has been gained and keep it off. I am confident that we will still have the weight off in two years.

We have been really amazed at the "eat as much as you like" principle. That's been a little difficult to accept because, intuitively, it just seems completely backwards to someone trying to lose weight—especially if you have tried so many other weight loss plans over the years that talk about consuming less food. When we first started *Let's Do Lunch* we only partially embraced this way of thinking. It wasn't until we fully embraced it that we understood and believed that this was real and could be a practical way of living.

We are excited to see new recipes on the chat boards at www.letsdolunch.com, and we check in frequently. . .

We also want you to know that we have two young children—ages 3 and 6—who are eating healthier since we started *Let's Do Lunch.* —K. K., CALIFORNIA

My point in sharing these three letters with you is that this is not just a fad diet plan to lose pounds. The plan *will* help you lose pounds—lots of pounds. But it's more than that. It's a way to better health. I don't know all the scientific reasons for this, but I know what works.

Through the years I've discovered that there are a large number of thin people who have adopted the *Let's Do Lunch* way of eating—not because they need to lose weight, but because they feel better eating the *Let's Do Lunch* way.

I could share dozens upon dozens of letters with you that tell amazing stories of weight loss. I will share a few notes and letters throughout the book, but the most amazing story is one that I know extremely well. It's *my* story, and that's where I'll begin.

At the outset, let me encourage you that you *can* turn things around. You *can* succeed even if you have failed dozens of times before in losing weight and keeping it off. You *can* do the *Let's Do Lunch* program and get thin.

I feel confident this plan will work for you. I feel confident that after you've been on the *Let's Do Lunch* program for a while, and get used to the eating changes, you will find that it becomes easier rather than harder. I firmly believe that once you've read and used the ideas in this book, you'll never think of eating any other way! There is no better motivation than seeing the weight loss you achieve on your scale. Once you have lost weight, please do me the favor of going to our Web site message boards and posting your success story there . . . and please don't thank me. Just privately give thanks to our Father and Jesus in heaven, and think about giving a love offering wherever there are people in need.

But before I get started with My Story, I want to say again that you must *trust* the plan. To begin with, you must eat until full whenever you are hungry, no matter how often that is and no matter how many calories you consume (even if you start by eating 10,000 calories a day). You must trust that by eating *Let's Do Lunch* foods, your blood sugar will stabilize, and your body will *force* you to become less hungry with each passing day.

I also want you to understand why I wrote this new edition of the book and why I made so many changes and additions to the original edition.

Let's Do Lunch has been a work in progress since I started losing weight in October of 1988. And quite frankly, until recently I really didn't understand why it worked. I knew it worked but not why.

When my wife and I started doing TV interviews, I remember telling interviewer after interviewer that *Let's Do Lunch* foods and recipes are just not fattening . . . that you can eat them until full, no matter how many calories you consume, and still lose weight. Each and every interviewer was very polite, but needless to say, I got some very strange looks!

Then during an interview in Houston, Texas, the interviewer challenged me by saying it was impossible to put unlimited calories in your body each and every day and still lose weight. My response was simply, "Well, here we are, living proof, and there are thousands of others who will tell you the same thing."

This new edition needed to be written if for no other reason than to explain why the program works.

Because of the input from many *Let's Do Lunchers*, as I call them, the ease with which you can lose weight has dramatically increased over the years. And for that reason, too, this new edition needed to be written.

For example, while I was writing this, I heard from a man who lost 83 pounds in his first three months on the plan. That is far more weight loss than the norm of 5 to 10 pounds a month, and he made his weight loss easier by doing two things that were not written in the previous edition of the book:

1. When eating each meal, he starts by eating half of what he normally eats. Then he takes a 10-minute break, during which time he drinks an 8 oz. glass of water. After that, he goes back to finish the rest of his meal . . . the benefit being he generally can't finish it. As he does this day after day, you can certainly understand how he has accelerated his weight loss.

2. He eats his heavy-protein meal at breakfast. Then he fills up on everything, except heavy proteins at *Let's Do Lunch* and at dinner. He says his heavy-protein breakfast holds him over for the rest of the day. In other words, he eats steak, chicken, turkey, and so forth for breakfast, and then he abstains from heavy proteins the rest of the day.

I absolutely love what he is doing in number 1, but I am *not* suggesting anyone try what works for him in number 2; I don't think that will work for most people.

Added to all of this, Let's Do Lunchers have also come up with several inventive and great-tasting recipes that fit in with the other staple recipes of the plan and warrant inclusion in this new edition. In other words, they are recipes that Let's Do Lunchers will eat over and over again, and they replace recipes from previous editions not of the staple ilk.

Further, new acceptable foods have become available over the years and can be eaten day in and day out instead of previous *Let's Do Lunch* foods that were allowed only occasionally.

Add to this the fact that better-tasting foods have also become available, and you have three more reasons for this new edition.

And finally, because of questions from previous-edition readers, many clarifications are also included in this new edition.

Now, on to how it all started back in 1988 . . . My Story

My Story

It Might Be Your Story Too!

As a little kid, my favorite thing to do was to go to Smitty's restaurant in La Porte, Indiana, and order a mouthwatering hamburger, deliciously greasy French fries, and an extra-thick chocolate "frosty malt." At every opportunity I ended up in a booth at Smitty's with one of my friends. I always felt a little mesmerized in anticipation of the food to come.

My parents knew about my fixation for this food, of course, and almost every Saturday night after Dad's gig (he had a band) they would wake me up by waving one of Smitty's burgers under my nose. I will remember as long as I live how terrific it was to wake up to this scent. This act of love endeared me to my mother and father forever.

Then came my downfall. To reward me for having brought home a good report card, my parents asked if there was anything special I would like. I thought about this for a while and decided I would like them to take me to Smitty's for "all I could eat." They agreed, and I proceeded to take in so many burgers, fries, and frosty malts that upon walking outside I upchucked all over the sidewalk. This was not what Mom and Dad had expected—nor had I—and looking back, it should have been a clue, but it wasn't.

A tradition started that night. Every time I did something good—such as make the basketball team, not miss any school, get up in the morning without being called a second time—I would ask my parents to take me to Smitty's to "pig out." It was what I wanted, and they consented. Food became a reward for me. This was the beginning of my addiction to food. Food brought pleasure. And if a little food brought a little pleasure, then more food brought more pleasure.

I ate like a horse and would assuredly have become as big as one if I hadn't been involved in athletics. Because of sports involvement, I kept my weight fairly stable and within bounds until I left college. After I married my wife, Anita, I stopped working out every day and became the proverbial couch potato. Unfortunately, my eating habits did not slow down. I gained weight by the week.

The fact that I was depressed because we were very poor didn't help matters. At my lowest moment, I remember Anita trying to cheer me up with the only thing that seemed to give me pleasure—besides her. She surprised me with two family-size pizzas she had purchased with the last money we had to our names—six valuable silver dollars that had been handed down to her, generation after generation. I cried, and she hugged me and stroked my hair and told me how much she loved me.

I rationalized my food addiction. I only ate when I was happy, sad, satisfied, frustrated, focused, confused, anxious, contented, encouraged, depressed, confident, afraid, or loving. The truth is I never ran out of reasons for eating. Within two years I had gained one hundred pounds.

I ate almost nonstop, from the time I got home from work until I went to bed. I ate everything you can imagine: hamburgers, hot dogs, tacos, nachos with cheese, French fries, milk shakes, sub sandwiches, fried chicken, fried fish, cheesecake, ice cream, chocolate bars, cashews—name any food that sounds good to the average person and I was a consumer of it!

I also ate throughout my workdays. I remember innumerable business luncheons when I actually told the waitress to serve me two full meals, one right after the other. I don't have to tell you how often my expense account was questioned.

Even Embarrassing Moments Didn't Keep Me from Stuffing My Face

Over the years, I paid a painful price for my compulsive overeating. Eating was fun, but being fat was not. I remember going to the "big and tall" clothing store and praying they had something in my size. I had a five-foot waist and a twenty-two-inch neck, and many times the shop simply didn't have anything in its inventory to fit me. I felt like a freak. When I flew first class and the stewardess had to bring me a seat belt extension, I was so embarrassed that I put my face in a magazine for the whole trip.

Then there were the times we went out to eat and everyone wanted to sit in a booth, but I just wouldn't fit. I could see the looks on the faces of the people around us as they snickered and whispered about my weight. I can't begin to tell you how bad I hurt when this happened. But I just couldn't help myself, I still sat down at a table and stuffed my big fat face.

It seems like yesterday that after I drove a golf cart, everyone in the clubhouse stared at the long black mark on my shirt caused by the steering wheel rubbing against my enormous belly. After I noticed the stares, I sat with my arms crossed over the mark and then sneaked out the back door. I went home feeling totally lost as to what to do about my problem.

I also remember my embarrassment at an amusement park, when everyone watched as I could not lock myself into the roller coaster and had to get up and leave. I went off by myself, unable to hold back the tears.

There was a day when I had to sit on one side of our friends' boat while everyone else sat on the other side. I didn't say a word as I anxiously awaited the end of the ride, and I never accepted an invitation like that again.

At a University of Minnesota wine-tasting party for the benefit of the Williams Scholarship Fund, I won the drawing for "your weight in wine." The master of ceremonies was stunned when he saw how much I weighed, but I was the one who was stunned when he announced to everyone, "The winner weighs 360 pounds!" I wanted to crawl under a table. I know my face turned beet red as I walked to the podium. That was the first time I had heard my weight broadcast to a roomful of people. The obvious now had a number attached to it, but that didn't keep the number from climbing higher.

Even when I least expected it, my weight caused me humiliation. My doctor—Neil Hoffman of Minneapolis, Minnesota—put me in the hospital for three days to give me a thorough physical. The very first evening as I was lying on my bed, I heard a loud, squeaky noise coming down the hall. Closer and closer it came to my room. Finally the door swung open as two nurses, both soaked in perspiration, wheeled in the hospital freight scale and asked me to please get on. I felt like a steer going to market. At that moment, I actually hated myself.

I lost all the weight I needed to lose, and I am still eating the way you taught me. I usually stay around 135 pounds, wear all the clothes I have wanted to wear, and I think I look pretty darn good. My eating has become such a habit that I forget sometimes that I'm actually doing *Let's Do Lunch*. It doesn't seem right if I have to eat dinner at dinner. I like it better at lunch, and am now teaching the young girl I work with how to eat. You made my life completely turn around, and I can't thank you enough.—*S.S., FLORIDA*

It Wasn't that I Didn't Try to Get
a Handle on Things . . .

Although my eating was out of control, I desperately tried again and again to get a handle on it. I attempted so many diets that it almost became funny to me, so much so that I went around telling my friends I was going to write a book called *How to Gain and Maintain, by R. T. Wilson, President of the Tons of Fun Weight Club.* I told people I would write pearls of wisdom, such as, "You must have chocolate during sex in order to make up for the calories being burned," and "Hamburgers are a must at the end of a gourmet evening because you'll still be starving."

Humor was a mask for my heavy-heartedness.

I was a professional dieting failure. I just didn't have the discipline and willpower necessary to succeed. In recent years I've discovered that many people have tried some of the same things I tried:

I Measured and Weighed

For about two weeks, I followed a diet that involved measuring and weighing food, food exchanges, and a weekly weigh-in and meeting. The problem was that I just didn't feel like I got enough to eat. Even though this program undoubtedly works for a lot of people, it didn't work for me.

I Tried High Protein and Fat

I ate cheese, bacon, eggs, meat, butter, and so forth, and lost some weight over a few weeks. But even though it worked in the short run, I got sick of eating all the greasy food that was prescribed and not being able to eat other foods. So, I gradually started eating in my old way and ended up heavier than I was before.

I Tried a Liquid Diet

I drank powders mixed in water and learned about nutrition. Once again, even though this program undoubtedly works for a lot of people, it just didn't work for me. I lasted about three weeks, until at a University of Minnesota basketball game I told my wife I felt very weird, like I was in a twilight zone. She said, "Forget it. This diet might be causing more harm than it's worth." I was off and eating again.

I'm a 60-year-old woman who has struggled with weight for the last 25 years. I have been on every diet plan known to mankind, counted calories, journaled points, exercised until I was ready to drop, was always hungry, prayed, cried, and had lost hope. Your plan has been a Godsend to me. I have been eating as you suggest for 3 weeks and have lost 10 pounds. My blood pressure has dropped around 15 points. I'm not hungry. The plan has fit into my busy schedule very well. I don't even think about food until mealtime.   —S. M., SOUTH DAKOTA

I Tried Acupuncture

I got to a point where I was desperate and willing to try just about anything. I went with our daughter's mother-in-law to an acupuncture specialist who stuck needles in our heads. This was supposed to cure her smoking problem and, of course, my weight problem. On our way home from the treatment, we looked at each other and burst out laughing. She lit up a cigarette and drove me to the doughnut shop.

I Tried the "Taste Only" Method

I decided it was only necessary to *taste* the foods I liked. So, without anyone knowing about it, I went to McDonald's and bought three Quarter Pounder burgers with cheese, two large orders of fries, two chocolate shakes, a cherry pie, and an apple pie. I then went into my bedroom and proceeded to chew the food but not swallow anything. That's right, I used an airline bag to deposit the food into after I had tasted it. The method didn't work, by the way. It lasted just that one meal.

Then Along Came a Very Good Reason to Lose Weight . . .

After a string of failures, along came a very good reason to lose some weight. Our daughter, Tyra, set a wedding date, and nothing had ever motivated me more to lose weight. And nothing I had done before or have done since was more painful than losing the weight I lost in order to proudly walk her down the aisle. I agonizingly pushed myself away from the table for nine months and got down to 278 pounds. I was so proud of myself! But the day of the wedding, even as I was walking her down the aisle, all I could think about was pigging out at the reception.

Can you imagine not being able to fully enjoy your own daughter's wedding because your mind is preoccupied with a vision of foods you have felt deprived of? That night I ate and drank everything in sight. I was off and eating again, and I gained back all the weight I had lost—plus more.

A Pattern of Monday Morning "Fresh Starts" Kicked In

Then—play it again, Sam—I got sick of the way I looked, and almost every Monday I'd start dieting again. I tried desperately to duplicate what I had done in losing weight for Tyra's wedding. By Monday night, my mind was tormented with thoughts of food.

The Monday-morning resolve lasted sometimes a day, sometimes two or three days, and then I would offer Anita or our son, Ty, money to go get a family-size pizza, lots of tacos and nachos with cheese, cashews, chocolate covered peanuts, chips and dip, cake, ice cream, chocolate bars—you name it and I bribed a member of my family to get it for me.

After gorging myself until I couldn't eat anymore, I would say to my wife, "Throw all the rest of this stuff away because I'm starting my diet tomorrow." Starting a diet the next day, of course, never happened. Anita got smart and refused to throw away the food. Instead, she would hide it from me so that when I asked for it again she would already have it and wouldn't have to spend additional money.

Anita tells me today that the reason she always went to the store to get what I wanted was simply that even though it hurt her terribly, she couldn't stand for me to be unhappy.

In my later fat years, because of all my embarrassments and humiliations, I became a "closet eater." When eating out, I would eat just like everyone else, and when I got home I would satiate myself with everything fattening I could get my hands on.

I started a little over a year ago. I've almost lost 85 lbs. and 5 sizes so far. I look so good that nobody believes I still have 50 more pounds to lose. My dad has lost 35 and he still uses it as his maintenance diet. —G. S., OHIO

Why Am I Willing to Tell You All This?

Why am I willing to admit all of this to you? Because no matter where you are on the dieting treadmill—trying again and again to lose weight, but instead of losing, you are gaining and gaining weight—there's a good chance I've "been there, done that." I know the pain, the humiliation, the temptations, and all the tricks of the dieting life.

But—and this is a huge, huge, huge turnaround statement for me—*I'm not fat today. I haven't been fat for years!* What happened?

I came to a very simple decision. I cried out to my Father in heaven and asked for help, and He answered my prayer. He gave me a plan that worked for *me*. I have spent several pages telling you what did not work for me, all to lead up to this point where I can tell you that I found something that does work for me. And since I'm something of an expert on what does *not* work, I hope you will see the wisdom in my sharing with you what does.

I developed a dieting plan that

- allows me to eat until I'm full.
- allows me to eat foods we all love.
- allows me to eat whenever I'm hungry.
- does not require that I do anything I hate to do.

Which means there's no exercising. There are no pills to take, no shakes to down, no counting of carbs, calories, fat grams, or points. There are no math exercises—no converting grams to calories. There's no measuring or weighing food, and no portioning. There are no prescribed foods to buy, no chemicals to take, and no specific liquids to drink. There are no meetings to attend.

I lost 230 pounds by eating foods we all love until I was completely full and could not eat any more. And—to the best of my knowledge—I became the only formerly obese person in the world to have written a diet book and kept the weight off.

As I started losing weight, my wife couldn't believe I was losing while I was eating a great deal of food and not exercising. She actually thought there was something wrong with me. She thought I was physically sick. She eventually voiced her concern to me, but initially, she was so happy to see me happy that she said nothing.

For the First Time, I Loved the
Side Effects of Weight Loss

Always in the past, I had hated the side effects of weight loss: I had no energy. I felt consumed with temptation to eat the wrong things. I was frustrated and depressed. This time, things were different. Almost immediately, I noticed major changes in my health—all of them positive.

My lower blood pressure number went from 90 and higher down to between 60 and 80. I got rid of my sleep apnea and snoring. My hips and feet stopped hurting. My acid indigestion left me. My face became thinner without any major sagging of the skin. My potassium level rose naturally. My skin stayed soft and smooth.

And most amazing to me, my waistline shrank even though I was eating until I was completely full. Because my cravings were eliminated, I didn't eat as much as I did before. I developed what I believe is the only way to speed up the body's metabolism naturally—without exercising, pills, and chemicals. I also found that it didn't matter where I ate my food. I ate lots of meals while lying on my bed, on my side.

As I mentioned before, Anita continued to fear that I was physically sick.

After I had lost approximately 190 pounds without exercising, she finally concluded that I must have cancer—that a major illness was the reason for my weight loss. She insisted that I have a thorough physical exam. I went to our dear friend, Dr. Eli Farri of Fort Myers, Florida, and he pronounced that I was fine and sent me home to tell Anita that whatever I was doing, I should continue doing it.

Anita cried. Shortly after that, she said, "Honey, please don't lose any more weight; you look just perfect." I can't begin to tell you how proud I felt!

I realize that you may not be a drinker, but I feel I need to say something to those who do drink. Until this time in my weight loss, I had completely abstained from drinking alcohol. Then, with Anita's pronouncement that I looked perfect and shouldn't lose any more weight, I decided to start drinking socially again. I decided to drink only wine. Even with these added calories, I lost another 40 pounds.

In retrospect, I realize that weight loss is more dramatic when alcohol is eliminated. I also maintain that it is not necessary to completely abstain in order to lose weight. If you drink wine, you will lose weight more slowly, but you will still lose on my plan.

After I lost the 230 pounds I wanted to lose, Anita was astounded and insisted I have another physical. Dr. Farri had to call and assure her there was nothing wrong with me. I don't have to tell you how pleased she was at that news. She looked at me as if I were the most wonderful China doll she had ever seen.

> To date I have dropped 58 pounds. I cannot believe how simple and painless this has been for me. I started slowly. I have read diet books before, but a life plan this simple? I lost 11 pounds just by eating frozen grapes for snacks! . . . People see me and cannot believe how I look. —B.M., FLORIDA

Then a Most Amazing Thing Happened

And then a most amazing thing happened—Anita asked me if I thought she could lose eight pounds on the program I had started calling "Let's Do Lunch." These eight pounds were ones she had not been able to lose all of her adult life. She didn't believe she could eat all the foods I told her she could eat and still lose weight, but she was willing to try. To make a long story short, Anita didn't lose eight pounds—she lost twenty-three pounds and is thinner now than she was at age eighteen!

After watching me eat to my heart's content one day, my mother said, "Honey, have you gone off your diet?" I told her that the way I was eating was the way I always ate on my diet, and I then asked if she was interested in losing any weight. She started doing the *Let's Do Lunch* plan and lost fifty pounds. She went from a dress size eighteen to a size ten, without exercise of any kind!

No, I'm Not a Movie Star—but Yes, I Am Your Cousin!

I told you about some of the most embarrassing experiences I had when I was heavy. Now I'd like to tell you about some of the fun experiences I've had as a thin man.

The foremost occasions that come to mind—some of them a little embarrassing and yet very gratifying for me—are the times people have thought I was a movie star or a TV personality. The first time this happened was in a restaurant in Louisville, Kentucky. Anita and I noticed everyone staring at us. Then the manager walked up, excused himself for interrupting, and said he recognized my face but couldn't remember my name. I told him I was sorry, but I didn't recall ever having met him. He said we'd never met, but he'd seen me in the movies and on television. I told him I was flattered, but I wasn't who he thought I was. He refused to hear my answer.

Instead, he said he understood my not wanting to be bothered, but he just wanted to thank us for dining at his restaurant. He told us we'd made his day, and he hoped we would enjoy ourselves enough to come back and see him again. I didn't know what to say, so I just thanked him for the kind words and told him if we ever came back to Louisville we would definitely stop and say hello. I was partly embarrassed, but partly ecstatic.

Then there was the episode at the jam-packed movie studio amusement park, when the casting director for their mock TV show selected our son, Ty, to be the announcer. I remember Ty looking at me and winking, as if to say, "Ha, ha, Dad, I got the part!" Then, right after he went through the dressing room door to prepare for the skit that was to follow, the casting director selected me to be the "leading man, main guest."

As I entered the dressing room, Ty looked up at me in astonishment and said, "What are you doing here?" When I told him, he just shook his head in disbelief—and *he* has never heard the end of it.

I remember calling three of my old working buddies to arrange a luncheon. I drove to downtown St. Paul, and as I was parking my car, I saw one of them doing the same. I didn't say a thing as we walked side by side into the restaurant. He had looked right at me and had no idea who I was! I turned toward him and asked if he had a match. Actually, I have no idea why I asked for a match, since I don't smoke. He replied that he did not. I said, "Well, you really ought to have a match for one of your old best buddies."

He looked at me again and stared. At last, he recognized me. His mouth dropped open. He was absolutely speechless. Finally, he threw his arms around me as he said, "I don't believe it!" It was all I could do to hold back the tears.

Even my best friend from high school didn't recognize me. When I arranged to meet him at a California hotel, my wife, my parents, and I arrived early and sat where we could see everyone coming in, but they could not see us. When my pal arrived, I got up and walked toward him. We looked at each other, and he continued walking right past me. I turned around and followed him.

He was obviously looking for me in the lobby, but when he didn't see the "old" me, he proceeded to a pay phone to make a call. I stood a few feet away and stared. He dropped his eyes to avoid my gaze and placed his call. When he looked up and saw that I was still staring at him, he said, "Is there something I can help you with, sir?" I said, "Well, you could help me find my best high-school buddy."

After what I said registered, his expression changed to shock, and he dropped the phone. He was speechless as he threw his arms around me. We joined my wife and my parents and talked and talked and talked. Several times during the conversation, he stopped just to stare at me. I felt as if I had won the lottery.

I've known Roger Troy Wilson for many years. I saw what he did with his weight. When he informed me about how he did it, I decided to give it a try. His program includes foods I liked, and I could eat amounts that satisfied my hunger. I lost 33 pounds and will continue eating this way because it is easy and rewarding.
—B. R., MINNESOTA

Blood relatives, too, didn't recognize me. While between flights at the Cleveland airport, I heard a voice I recognized. I said, "Shelly?" The woman looked at me, and when she didn't recognize me, she somewhat reluctantly said, "Yes." I just stared at her, and she stared back. "Do I know you?" she finally asked.

I said, "Well, you should—I've been your cousin since you were born." She stared at me for the longest time and finally said, "Roger Troy?" I said, "Yes," and she threw her arms around me and screamed. Several times during the conversation that followed, she looked at me and lost her train of thought. I had to pry myself away in order to catch my plane. When I reached the gate, I turned around and there she was. She had followed me and just stood there in a daze. Later, I found out she called family members across the country to tell them I looked like a movie star! Boy, were my buttons popping when I heard about that.

Imagine how I felt the first time I attended my high-school class reunion sporting a svelte body—especially since I had been progressively heavier at each of the previous ones. As Anita and I planned, I walked into the room alone. People were looking at me, wondering who I was. Finally, one classmate came over and asked if I was the guest speaker. Absolutely no one had an inkling as to my identity. What a commotion I caused! And what an absolutely marvelous time I had showing off my thinness and dancing with my old girlfriends. I was the talk of the town.

By now you have probably wondered if any problems resulted from my incredible weight loss. There was only one: I had an apron of skin hanging from my tummy. Even though I could have lived with it the rest of my life, I chose to have a tummy tuck. I interviewed several plastic surgeons and selected Dr. William Carter of Edina Plastic Surgery, in Edina, Minnesota. I must admit I was a bit surprised when he told me that he was going to need to cut approximately 50 percent of the way around my body because of my previous massive size.

In addition to removing the excess skin, Dr. Carter also tightened all the muscles in my stomach. Upon viewing his masterpiece, he looked at his nurse and said, "Look at that—he looks like a twenty-five-year-old!" I have absolutely never, ever been so happy about anything in my life! To have a board for a tummy, after living with a five-foot waist, is the most triumphant feeling you can imagine.

The Best News of All Wasn't Related to My Looks

The best part of being thin, of course, was not in the compliments or "surprises" related to my appearance. It came in another form. Prior to my tummy tuck, I needed a medical examination to ensure that I was physically able to have surgery. My friend, Dr. Neil Hoffman of Minneapolis, Minnesota, performed the pre-op exam.

A few days after surgery, I received the following letter from Dr. Hoffman:

Dear Roger:

I hope the surgery went well. I just wanted to let you know that your blood count was normal, your urinalysis looked good, and your cholesterol is 158. *Tell Anita the bad news is this means you're going to live a long time.* All your blood fats look good. Your blood sugar, liver, kidney, and bone function studies are normal. So just a quick note to let you know that all of your laboratory studies including your coagulation studies, thyroid, blood fats all look normal and that I hope things went well. I look forward to seeing you again.

Most sincerely,

Neil R. Hoffman, M.D., F.A.C.P.

Nothing can beat the good news of a great health report!

Are You Wondering Just How I Lost So Much Weight?

I can hardly wait to tell you. It all began with a few bunches of grapes. But before I begin, I want you to know that *Let's Do Lunch* is not a fruit diet! In fact, if you never eat or crave desserts, candy, or other sweets, then you don't need to eat any fruit at all—just do the rest of the *Let's Do Lunch* program. Likewise, if there is any food you don't like, just leave it out. And please read chapters 2 through 6 at least three times. That said . . .

Grapes

And More Glorious Grapes

I'll always remember that fateful day when my life was changed forever. I remember it like it was yesterday. It was a beautiful October night, and I was in my summer home in Minneapolis, watching TV. I decided—as was usual for me in my 425-pound state—that it was "pig-out time." So, for the fifteen-thousandth time in my life, I went to the kitchen to find something to eat. I was in search of cookies and coffee, or cake and ice cream, or a big frozen chocolate bar. Something sweet. Something delicious.

I opened the freezer and, to my surprise, I found several very large bunches of grapes. They were ruined—frozen solid! I accused Anita of ruining perfectly good grapes by putting them in the freezer, but she said she didn't do it.

Aha! The culprit had to be our son, Ty. I blame him for everything even if he's not in town. I called Ty at the Billiard Street Cafe in Fridley, Minnesota—he and his partner own the place. I said, "Hey, Son, when you're over at our house, please have the common courtesy not to ruin our food."

Ty told me in very direct terms that the grapes were *not* ruined. He said that I obviously had never eaten frozen grapes—

they were a great snack food, they had the texture of a Popsicle, and freezing the grapes enhanced their sweetness. He concluded by telling me that frozen grapes were much better for me than all the garbage I normally ate.

I didn't believe a word of it—or perhaps I did. I decided for some reason to try one. I loved it! It was cold, made my mouth feel good, and somehow freezing did enhance the sweetness. Thank you, Son.

I ate frozen grapes until my mouth was numb. I decided I didn't want any more. It is important that you understand what I'm saying. I literally ate so many grapes that I was sick of them and just couldn't eat any more. I'm talking pounds of them. Thousands of calories of them!

I wandered to the kitchen to get something *else* to eat— maybe some chips and dip, or maybe a family-size pizza. But lo and behold, I discovered I didn't *want* anything else. This had never happened before. I wasn't hungry, so I went to bed.

The next evening *exactly* the same thing happened! That's when I decided to eat frozen grapes every night—instead of junk food—while watching TV. After about a month of this new habit, I noticed some of my clothes were loose. I obviously had lost a few pounds even though I was eating thousands of calories of frozen grapes each night, and even though I was still drinking and eating in my same old fattening way at dinnertime.

I've been following the program now for about seven months and my clothes fit again! I can buy normal sizes—I was a 48, I'm now a 40. I feel just great! It's a fun program, something you really CAN live with. —*W. M., PENNSYLVANIA*

As I mentioned earlier, I want you to understand one very important thing: *Let's Do Lunch is not a fruit diet!* This is not a "grape" diet. Grapes may be included in the program, but for me, this discovery of frozen grapes was just the *beginning*. The *Let's Do Lunch* plan *also* includes burgers, steaks, baked beans, corn on the cob, barbecue chicken, glazed salmon, Caesar salads, omelets, sloppy joes, stuffed peppers, chicken Parmesan, chili, tuna salad, meatloaf, and many other foods you probably would never think of eating while trying to lose weight.

Don't worry if you can't tolerate, or simply don't like, certain fruits. You choose the fruits you eat—as well as how much you eat—and you can eat canned fruits. If you have physical problems, such as colitis or diabetes, see your doctor for a list of fruits that are best for you.

Further, let me shock you a little. After fifteen years of experimenting with my own body and diet program, it is my firm belief that fruit sugar (fructose) is *not* fattening—no matter how many calories are involved. I have come to an unshakable opinion that refined and processed sugars are extremely fattening even though they have no fat grams in them. But fruit itself, and the sugar that is in fruit, is not fattening.

After I figured out I could eat pounds of frozen grapes every evening and lose weight, I started to wonder whether I could eat oodles of other fruits and lose weight. So, I started eating as much as I wanted of all different kinds of fruits in place of my normal evening junk food. I ate mangos, kiwifruit, watermelon, cantaloupe, melon, strawberries, pears, apples, plums, honeydew, oranges, tangerines, peaches, and, of course, grapes. To give you an idea of the volume of fruit I ate, at one sitting I consumed half a watermelon, a whole cantaloupe, four tangerines, four plums, two apples, and then finished with a pound of grapes. And I lost weight.

I was on a roll! I was losing weight, and it was easy!

Because I was losing weight and didn't feel the least bit deprived, I had a growing desire to lose weight even faster. I started thinking about eliminating all the fattening foods and drinks I was eating at mealtimes. You know, just eat veggies, soups, salads, lean meat, chicken, turkey, and fish from that point on. Of course, I had tried that many times before—unsuccessfully. The sad fact is that most of these foods tasted awful when prepared in a dietary way. I was just *thinking* about this at the time. I hadn't taken any steps to actually eliminate any foods.

Then I awoke in the middle of the night with an idea: if I didn't like something that was nonfattening, why not add a little something to make it taste great? It was worth a try.

Another major point: *Let's Do Lunch is* not *all about cutting back on fat grams and calories.*

On this plan you can eat *all the carbs you want,* along with proteins and fats—and lose weight. Furthermore, you can lose weight without suffering cravings of any kind. This program incorporates all of the food groups: meats, starches, fruits, vegetables, dairy, and fats. There is no elimination of any food group or meal. This is one of the major reasons for the plan's success. You aren't limited to any particular type of food.

I developed seven strategies of eating. Frozen grapes and a host of other fruits were my snack foods.

7 Strategies that Really Worked for Me

Remember that I was thinking about eating the foods that I knew were "right" for dieting, but was also thinking about adjusting the way I ate those foods so that I would like them. Following are seven strategies that worked for me as I first began to lose weight and to develop the *Let's Do Lunch* plan.

Strategy #1: I "Leaned Up" My Meat.

I discovered that if I mixed extra-lean hamburger and skinless ground turkey or chicken breast together, the turkey or chicken took on the flavor of the beef, and I could not tell the difference. I could eat regular portions of "burgers" and have less fat. I put some mashed pinto beans and chopped onions into the beef and turkey or chicken mixture before I formed the patties. I fried these in a nonstick pan I coated with extra-virgin olive oil cooking spray. Delicious! I ate to my heart's content, dipping my fork into on-the-side ketchup, mustard, relish, and onions—and I lost weight.

LET'S DO LUNCH BURGERS . . . delicious, and eat them as often as you want!

½ lb. lean ground sirloin
½ lb. ground turkey or chicken breast (skinless)
1   cup finely chopped onions
1   16 oz. can pinto beans, drained

Mash pinto beans and mix with ground turkey or chicken and ground sirloin and onions. Season with salt and pepper. Make into patties (use egg white to hold them together if necessary). Spray pan or grill with olive oil spray. Fry or grill. Serve with your favorite condiments. Make a double batch, and store in freezer.

As a variation, I made chili with half extra-lean ground beef and half skinless ground turkey or chicken breast. Outstanding! Three or four large bowls normally did the trick—and I lost weight. I even developed a way to make chicken or turkey taste like beef (see recipe for Edna Ruth's Chicken or Turkey in chapter 9).

Strategy #2: I Made Fish Enjoyable.

I like fish, but I don't like it plain. So I grilled, broiled, baked, or blackened fish. But then I dipped my fork into on-the-side tartar sauce—just enough so the tines of the fork were covered for each bite or so of fish. I made this sauce myself with some sweet relish and Hellmann's Reduced Fat cholesterol-free mayonnaise. Fish was delicious with this strategy—and I ate all the fish I wanted and still lost weight. It is important that you understand what I just said: I didn't eat just three and a half ounces of grilled or blackened fish. Sometimes—actually, most of the time—I ate three or four whole fillets.

Strategy #3: I "De-lettuced and Blue-cheesed" My Salad.

I prepared a salad that had a three-bean salad at the base. On top of this I put peas, corn, onions, tomatoes, beets, green peppers, and a small amount of my all-time favorite cheese—blue cheese. I dipped my fork into a little dish of reduced-calorie French dressing or a Newman's Own dressing. I loved this salad. It's *great*! And once more, I ate all I wanted and still lost weight.

LET'S DO LUNCH DE-LETTUCED SALAD WITH AGED CHEESE . . . salads will never be the same again!

- 2   cups 3-bean salad, drained
- 1   cup peas, drained
- 1   cup corn, drained
- ½   cup pickled beets, drained
- ½   cup cut-up green pepper
- 1   cup diced onion
- 1   large tomato or 2 small tomatoes, cut up
- ½   cup of your favorite aged-cheese crumbles
      (My favorite is blue cheese.)

Mix together, and top with a small amount of your favorite no-fat or low-fat dressing. Make a double batch, and store in refrigerator.

Strategy #4: I Found Ways to Make Veggies More Interesting.

I found a vegetable dish I really liked. It involved a large package of mixed fresh veggies from the produce section of the store. After washing these and steaming them lightly, I melted two slices of cheese over the veggies in the microwave. I used Borden fat-free sharp nonfat processed cheese product. I loved eating veggies this way, and I ate all I wanted—and still lost weight.

Strategy #5: I Found a Favorite Meal.

Actually I found several favorite meals. One was meat and beans. I brought home hot barbecue chicken from the grocery store, took the skin off, and ate the meat and sauce with a three-bean salad from the deli section of the store. The salad was made with some oil, so I drained off the oil before eating. For lots of meals, I'd eat the whole chicken and a quart of three-bean salad, while my wife watched in astonishment! And I lost weight.

Strategy #6: I Became an Expert at Making a Veggie Omelet.

I frequently made a large omelet without cheese—but with tomatoes, green peppers, and onions. I ate it with salsa. Sometimes I'd savor a six-egg monstrosity. I could whip one of these up in just a couple of minutes.

Strategy #7: I Switched to Milk Instead of Cream in My Coffee.

I drank my coffee with skim milk instead of the cream I normally used. Over time, I not only got used to the lighter taste but preferred it. Then I switched from coffee to water—and at lunch, iced tea.

Are you getting the idea behind my strategies? I was eating *good* foods, but I was also making them *taste* good.

At this stage of the program, at meal times I was eating veggies, soups, salads, red meat, chicken, turkey, and fish. I drank and ate all I wanted. I was losing weight, my way.

My weight loss is slow, but I'm still losing and very grateful. The program has benefited me the most, however, with my diabetes. I have come down to where my blood sugar is about 100 or less, and my average for each month is 6.9 from nearly 10 HBLIC. Thanks! —*L. R., Oklahoma*

When I Wanted "Just a Little Something"

I then found that I didn't need a big meal every time I sat down to eat. Sometimes I wanted "just a little something." Here are two of my favorite quick and easy dishes:

- Store-bought, sliced, baked turkey, with a slice of Kraft fat-free cheese melted on it and served on a slice of Wasa Light Rye Original Crispbread. Wasa crispbread looks like a huge cracker and is fat free. I ate from one to four of these.

- Tuna salad, mixed with just enough Hellmann's reduced-fat cholesterol-free mayonnaise to hold it together. I put this on a slice of Wasa Light Rye Original Crispbread, along with fresh tomato, sweet relish, and onion. I ate from one to four of these.

Not Only Was I Losing Weight . . .

You'll note that I said repeatedly, "and I lost weight." I did! And here's what will blow your mind: my waistline shrank even though I was eating tremendous volumes of food. Over the course of the diet, my waistline shrank twenty-four inches. That's *two feet* around my middle!

Today, as I'm writing this, there is absolutely no way I could eat the volumes of food I ate when I first started *Let's Do Lunch*.

Because my blood sugar became stabilized, I became less hungry with each passing day. Thus, I began to eat less.

- The food tasted good.
- There was lots of variety.
- I didn't feel as if I was denying myself something special.
- I was dropping pounds.

And it was easier than anything I had ever done before.

Keep in mind that many distinguished people, including my family doctors, witnessed my weight loss.

You May Not Have a Mountain of Fat to Lose

You may be saying, "But Roger Troy, you had a mountain of fat to lose. I only want to lose a few pounds."

Remember that my own mother went from a size eighteen dress to a size ten dress on the program, without exercise of any kind.

My wife wanted to lose only eight pounds when she started the program. She had carried those extra eight pounds all of her adult life and had found them virtually impossible to lose. She's five feet seven inches tall, and she's never been overweight by other people's standards. But she wanted to lose eight pounds nonetheless. She was hesitant about even trying my program—simply because she saw me eating such large quantities of food. She couldn't fathom how she could possibly eat good-tasting food until she was full and still lose weight.

But finally she said to me, "Honey, do you think I could go on *Let's Do Lunch* and lose the eight pounds I've always wanted to lose?"

"What's the worst that can happen?" I asked her. "If it doesn't work for you, simply go back to what you have been doing. No harm, no foul."

She decided to try the *Let's Do Lunch* plan, and she didn't just lose the eight pounds—she lost twenty-three pounds!

This Was Just the Beginning . . .

These basics were just the beginning for me. Remember that I had 230 pounds to lose. But it was a great beginning! I figure any time you can eat foods you like that taste good, in quantities that are satisfying, and still lose weight—you're off to a good start.

Let me tell you the big secrets I learned to keep the weight rolling off. But before I do that, hot off the presses are the following new *Let's Do Lunch* foods:

- Dry Roasted Soy Nuts, no sugar added (mix with raisins and enjoy, or coat them in melted soy margarine, season with Konriko Jalapeno All Purpose Seasoning, spread them on a tray, and bake for 5 minutes at 400 degrees)
- Real Foods Original Corn Thins (some people like these better than Wasa Light Crispbread)
- Willow Run Soy Margarine (again, has a good taste when used in recipes and for cooking)
- Dark-brown Brown or Red Rice and Wild Rice (*no* light-colored brown rice)
- Fat Free Light Rye RY KRISP, whole rye, no sugar
- Original Shredded Wheat, 100% whole wheat, no sugar
- Quaker Multi-Grain Hot Cereal, whole grain, no sugar
- Popcorn-flour Pancakes, Butter-bean Potato Cakes, Ground-chicken Sausages, and Tomato Soup (see chapter 9)

Note: 71 Laminated Recipe Cards for $15 (order at www.letsdo lunch.com*)*

Now, on to the big secrets . . .

4 Big Secrets

And the Plan that Puts Them into Practice

The process of dropping 230 pounds was a fascinating one. Along the way, I experimented with lots of different things—especially different types of foods to see what effect they had on weight loss. I found some fattening foods to be non-fattening, and some so-called nonfattening foods to be fattening. I found that there were some fattening foods I just couldn't avoid. Along the way, I came to several conclusions that I call the "Big Secrets." They are the keys that make the *Let's Do Lunch* program so successful.

The Big Secrets Are the Keys to Success

The Big Secrets are the key concepts that came into sharp focus for me as I attempted to create a weight-loss plan that would work for *me*.

Big Secret #1: You Must Eat a Little Fruit Every Day.
At the beginning of the diet, you must eat enough fruit to kick your addiction to desserts, candy, and other sweets. You

need to eat as much fresh fruit—especially the sweetest fruits—
as you can possibly tolerate putting into your body each and
every day until you start to crave fruit instead of other sugars. It
is imperative that you eat fruit every time you have an urge for
anything sweet—no matter what time of day it is. You must keep
eating fruit until your sweet tooth is satisfied. After a while, you
will be able to get by on just a little fruit each day.

Big Secret #2: Make Lunch Your Main Meal of the Day, Except for the Days When Your Work Prevents It.

Limit your heavy protein intake to lunch. I'll present the full
program to you later in this chapter, but for now, get this secret
embedded in your mind: *Lunch is the main meal of the day!*

"But," you may be saying, "dinner . . ." I know. I know. Just
remember that dinner can remain your main protein meal. The
program has flexibility. But for every day that it is possible, you
must have your main protein-rich meal at lunch. And yes, you
can do this. There are lots of tips that will show you how.

Big Secret #3: Choose the Least Fattening Option that Tastes Good to You.

If you are faced with alternatives to satisfying a craving,
choose the least fattening item that tastes good to you. There's
no point in eating foods that you dislike or that taste like card-
board or Styrofoam. Eat foods you like and you'll stick with a
program forever. Eat foods you don't like, that don't taste good,
or that simply don't satisfy, and you'll chalk up one more dieting
failure.

"The least fattening that tastes the best" means that some
brands taste better than others. Occasionally a brand might have
a few less fat grams, but the brand simply didn't taste good to
me. I knew if I was going to eat anything on a continuing basis,
it had to taste great. I tried many brands to determine the ones

that I personally could label as "the least fattening that tastes the best." The shopping list chapter (chapter 8) and the recipe chapter (chapter 9) identify those specific brands.

If you don't like something I like, then find the least fattening alternative that tastes the best to you, and have at it.

Patti and I each lost 25 pounds in two months! We are so excited about this program—it really works and we don't even feel like we're dieting. In fact, we like *Let's Do Lunch* so much that we've given four books to friends already! —*R. B., ARIZONA*

Big Secret #4: Trade Out Bread, Pasta, Potatoes, and Rice for *Unprocessed* Beans, Corn, Peas, and Corn Thins.

I strongly believe that bread, pasta, potatoes, and rice are like eating cake. I believe that the *calories* assigned to these foods are bogus—because these foods turn into pure fat!

About a year into my diet, I went to the store to find the least fattening bread that tasted the best, and found an Italian bread with one-half gram of fat and sixty calories per slice that tasted terrific. I tested my theory by eating four slices of this bread with only a light layer of diet jam as my breakfast each morning, for two weeks. And what happened? My weight loss halted.

It wasn't possible, however, for me to give up bread completely. I love sandwiches. There were times when the only thing I wanted to eat was a sandwich. How could I have a tuna salad sandwich without having a slice of bread?

I decided that it wasn't necessary for me to have two slices of bread to have a sandwich. When I was eating out I'd simply have my sandwich served open-face on one slice of bread, and eat it with a fork. I'd order my sandwich on rye or whole-wheat bread. If a whole-grain bun was an option on the menu, I'd scoop out the inside of half of the bun and put the sandwich ingredients in that half. I discarded the other half and the scooped-out portion.

When I was at home, I ate crispbread (whole-grain, fat-free, and sugar-free) instead of bread. I ate as little as possible, but I did enjoy burgers, tuna salad, chicken salad, and soups with a little of this crispbread.

Other than that I tried to abstain from breads and crackers. This meant no rolls, buns, bagels, muffins, biscuits, croissants, crackers, bread sticks, flat bread, slices of bread, or breaded foods at mealtimes—or anytime for that matter.

Crispbreads are a processed food, and processed foods are not good for weight loss. Instead, eat Real Foods Original Corn Thins, which are pressed popcorn (amazon.com).

Unprocessed foods such as beans, corn, peas, and Corn Thins are wonderful. Always remember, eating unprocessed means losing weight. Eating processed means gaining weight.

On occasion—and certainly not often—I had some yolk-free egg noodles, which have fewer fat grams than other noodles. I'd top a small portion of noodles with generous portions of acceptable no-sugar spaghetti sauce or mixed veggies with a slice or two of fat-free sharp nonfat cheese melted on top. Or I'd eat as much as I wanted of Butter-bean Potato Cakes or Bill's Mashed Potatoes (see chapter 9). These recipes are delicious!

Other than these few items, I stayed away from bread, potatoes, pasta, noodles, and rice because I consider them breads. I also didn't eat waffles, pancakes, doughnuts, and other starchy grain foods—they, too, are breads.

If you crave cereal, then eat as little as possible, and choose ones that are whole grain and contain neither sugar nor cane juice, for example, Quaker Oats 100% Whole Grain Cereal. If you can, eat this cereal with hot water or fat-free skim milk and diet sweetener.

The great benefit of corn, peas, and beans. Some people consider beans, peas, and corn as fattening foods. These are starchy protein vegetables, but I firmly believe they are nonfattening and can be eaten in large quantities. I ate oodles of corn, peas, and beans in place of potatoes, pasta, bread, and other grain starches. These foods not only totally satisfied my need for bread, but—I lost weight! Try the Beef Recipes with beans in them!

A nutritionist recently told me that a half cup of beans has seven to nine grams of protein as well as sixteen to twenty-eight grams of carbohydrates. Most wheat products, in comparison, have two to three grams of protein and fifteen grams of carbohydrates. While eating beans I was eating more protein than if I had been eating grains. A potato has virtually no protein.

The great amount of vegetables and fruits in the *Let's Do Lunch* program provides lots of valuable vitamins and minerals to a person's overall eating plan, including a high quantity of potassium, folate, niacin, vitamin A, vitamins B6 and B12, vitamin C, minerals, and phytochemicals. So much for the nutritional science. Let me tell you about the experience.

In most cases, I found that I was very satisfied if I had a big variety of beans, peas, and corn, in addition to onions, tomatoes, mushrooms, and other vegetables that are not starchy and have no protein. I ate beans in my soups and chili. I ate peas and beans on my salads, and peas and corn in my mixed veggies. I found I liked tomato soup with acceptable mixed veggies in it—including beans, peas, and corn. I ate corn on the cob with olive oil sprayed on it. You can't imagine how great-tasting olive oil is when sprayed on corn and popcorn. My wife makes this in huge quantities—and she makes it often. A good friend and successful Let's Do Luncher, Mary Simmons, sent me a white-bean soup recipe that we have adopted as our own. I eat dozens upon dozens of bowls of this soup. Here is the recipe:

LET'S DO LUNCH BEAN SOUP . . .
you'll become addicted!

4   regular-size cans northern or navy beans, drained
1   cup chopped yellow onion
1   crushed or minced clove of garlic
1   Knorr chicken bouillon cube
1½ tsp. dried Mixed Italian Herbs or Herbes de
    Provence
1   tbsp. olive oil

Pour olive oil in a large saucepan with lid. When it is hot, add the onion and garlic. Sauté, stirring frequently, on medium-high for 3 minutes.

Add the beans. Mash mixture with potato masher. Bring to a boil. Add the bouillon cube, the herbs, and a bit of ground black pepper to taste. Stir well and reduce heat to medium-low. Add water for desired thickness. Cover and cook for 10 minutes.

One day I looked up the definition of *corn* in *Webster's New World Dictionary,* and here's what I found: "a small, hard seed or seed-like fruit"—and you already know what I think of fruit!

I also ate lots and lots of Orville Redenbacher's 94 percent fat-free popcorn—without butter on top, but sprayed with a 100 percent extra-virgin olive oil spray. My mother actually uses popcorn in place of bread, doing things like frying "eggs over easy" in olive oil and eating them with popcorn on top.

I found that by eating beans, peas, and corn in good quantity, I no longer had any cravings for breads, pasta, potatoes, cereals, noodles, and rice. That was as close to a miracle as a fat person can get. The reality is that most overweight people eat a lot of breads, pasta, potatoes, noodles, crackers, cereals, rice, waffles, pancakes, and doughnuts. If you are one of them, hear me loud and clear: *eat as many recipes with beans, corn, and peas as you can possibly tolerate—such as Bill's Mashed Potatoes.*

Remember, for weight loss, Real Foods Original Corn Thins are better than crispbreads (buy at a health-food store, amazon.com, or glutensmart.com). When buying whole-grain cereals, make sure there is no sugar or cane juice in the ingredients (for example, Original Shredded Wheat 100% Whole Wheat).

The *Let's Do Lunch* plan calls for you to try to eliminate eating potatoes, rice, and foods made from flour. This means no potatoes, rice, rolls, buns, bagels, pasta, noodles, crackers, and bread. In their place, you'll be eating high-fiber beans, corn, and peas as well as Corn Thins.

"But," you may be grimacing, "there's a problem with beans . . ." Yes, I know. And there's also a solution. It's called Beano. You can get it at your favorite health-food store and many grocery stores. For those who don't like beans, you can't even taste them in most of the recipes (chapter 9).

The Basics of
the *Let's Do Lunch* Plan

And now—drumroll—let's put the four Big Secrets into a daily eating plan. Here's where things get exciting. Following are the basics of the *Let's Do Lunch* program.

Breakfast

Eat as much fresh fruit as you want, such as a banana, an apple, a grapefruit. I lost weight faster when I ate grapefruit or had a fruit smoothie for breakfast. For some of you on blood pressure and some other medicines, physicians advise that you *not* eat grapefuit in any form. Be sure to check with your physician.

I found that fruit digests faster than other foods and therefore, if eaten by itself, it tends to speed up the body's metabolism naturally. If fresh fruit is not available, then eating canned or frozen fruit is okay. If only fruit juice is available, that's okay occasionally.

If you are a person who needs something more substantial for breakfast, keep reading, and also read the 14-Day Meal Guide in chapter 7. If you crave cereal for breakfast, eat only whole grain with no sugar or cane juice in the ingredients.

Then—if possible—eat nothing throughout the rest of the morning. In most cases, that will mean you are famished by lunchtime. That's good! Remember:

- Fresh fruits and a fruit smoothie at breakfast speed up your metabolism.
- Eat nothing the rest of the morning so you will have a big appetite at lunch.

Lunch

This is your big meal of the day. (For those people whose time prevents a big meal at lunch, switch this Lunch to Dinner. An explanation follows.)

At lunch, eat extra-lean red meat, chicken, turkey, fish, and other acceptable proteins (identified later), along with all you can eat of acceptable soups, salads, and vegetables.

You might eat lean steaks, lean hamburger, baked beans, corn on the cob, popcorn, barbecue chicken, glazed salmon, Caesar salads, omelets, tuna salad, chili, chicken Parmesan, beef stew, taco salad, barbecue beef, egg salad, bean soup, chicken salad, coleslaw, chicken chow mein, three-bean salad, stuffed peppers, or meatloaf. These are all healthy foods. And, you can eat them with all of the regular sauces and condiments, for example, ketchup, mustard, and tartar sauce.

It is imperative that you eat a generous portion of protein. Protein will keep you satisfied longer, so you don't get terrible cravings for snacks in the afternoon or become tempted to eat all the wrong foods at dinnertime.

If you are craving bread, pasta, rice, or potatoes at noon, be sure to eat some special salsa, antipasto, corn on the cob, popcorn, or something with corn, beans, or peas in it. That will eliminate the craving. Go for Bill's Mashed Potatoes.

After eating lunch, eat nothing more until dinnertime. Remember:

- Eat your only protein of the day at lunch.
- Do not snack in the afternoon.

I saw the newspaper ad for your book 17 months ago, ordered it, and gave it a try. I lost over 25 pounds and have successfully kept it off. It has changed the way I eat and the way I think about eating. My teenage daughters are eating better because of your book . . . Thank you for all you have done for me. You have changed my life. — *J. M., MARYLAND*

Dinner

For dinner, first eat as much as you can of fruit. Again, fresh fruit is much better for you, but if fresh is not available, then eat frozen or canned fruit. Once again, you'll be speeding up your metabolism. Sometimes I eat a banana, grapes, or frozen grapes. Eat until you are totally satisfied.

My favorite first thing to have at dinnertime was and is a "smoothie." Here's my basic smoothie recipe:

ROGER TROY'S SMOOTHIE

In a blender, blend 6 ice cubes with

- 1½ cups unsweetened orange, pineapple, or apple juice
- Half of a frozen banana
- Any other frozen or fresh fruit

Sometimes I substitute unsweetened frozen fruit for the ice cubes, and I may need to add a little water for the correct consistency. These drinks are very soothing and satisfying.

Note: Peel and cut bananas in half and put them in freezer bags.

If—and only if—you are not satisfied after having fruits or fruit smoothies for dinner, then you may eat acceptable soups, salads, vegetables, special salsa, antipasto, corn on the cob, popcorn, or something with beans, peas, or corn in it until you are satisfied. *But do not eat protein for dinner.* Remember:

- At dinner eat as much fruit as you can, preferably fresh, although canned or frozen fruit is acceptable.
- Try having fruit smoothies as your dinner.
- If a fruit or smoothie dinner doesn't satisfy you, eat other foods that are listed as acceptable—but *no protein.*

Occasionally people will tell me after they've been on the *Let's Do Lunch* plan for a while that they find a dinner of all fruit too sweet. My advice is to cut down on the amount of fruit. You may be satisfied with less fruit over a period of time.

Why no protein at night? Think about it: Which is better, lying dormant in bed all night with only fast-digesting, nonfattening foods to metabolize, or lying there with your stomach full of slow-digesting foods that will turn mostly to fat in a dormant body?

Evening Snacks

If you get the munchies during the late evening or even in the middle of the night, eat some fresh fruit or fruit salad, or have a second fruit smoothie. Anita and I keep a small box of Sun-Maid raisins on each of the end tables in our bedroom so we can satisfy our sweet tooth at any time.

There are other acceptable evening snacks listed in the 14-Day Meal Guide in chapter 7. If fruits or fruit smoothies just don't do it for you, then go for one of the other snacks I have mentioned within this book.

Switching Lunch to Dinner

There are many people whose time prevents a big protein meal at lunch. There are also days when for one reason or another, you don't have lunch at all. And, there are those special dinners where protein is served. On those days, switch your heavy protein meal to dinner.

On your "switch" days, eat *no fruit* and *no protein* at lunch— just eat acceptable soups, salads, vegetables, special salsa, antipasto, corn on the cob, popcorn, or something with beans, peas, or corn in it.

Then, just prior to having a protein-based dinner, eat all the fruit you can.

If you are attending a dinner party, eat the nonfattening foods and the proteins and say "no, thank you" to dessert.

Remember:

- When the regular *Let's Do Lunch* lunch is going to be eaten at dinnertime, eat *no fruit* and *no protein* at lunch—just eat other acceptable foods.
- Just before eating a protein dinner—your only protein of the day—eat all the fresh fruit you can.

Well, it's been around 7 months since Angela's story was on this website. . . . I'm happy to report that she is looking and feeling better than ever, thanks to *Let's Do Lunch*. Her main challenge was that her job would not allow her to switch around lunch for dinner, so she still has her main meal at night time rather than in the middle of the day. . . . Despite the challenge of having to eat her protein at night, she finally got out of maternity clothes around 5 months ago. Then, only three months later, she went and bought size 12 clothes, which is smaller than she has been for years. Angela has lost around 80 pounds total. We're all so happy for her! —M. S., *FLORIDA*

A Word About "All that Fruit"

I told you in the first few pages of this book that the *Let's Do Lunch* program is not a fruit diet. It isn't. It's a program that includes foods from all the food groups.

You may be questioning, however, the quantities of fruit I recommend. Let me assure you this is a healthy way to live for most people. In fact, Dr. Michael Criqui and others at the University of California, San Diego, Medical Center found in one of their scientific medical research studies that people who lived longest were those who ate the most fresh fruit. Granted, there are some people—such as those with colon diseases and diabetes—who may not be able to eat as much fruit as recommended here. Consult your physician. You may be able to eat more fruit of restricted types than you think. If your doctor says "no fruits of any kind," just do the rest of the *Let's Do Lunch* program—with your doctor's permission, of course.

I strongly believe that fructose—sugar from fruits—is not fattening. It is *processed* sugars (glucose and sucrose and all of the various syrups and processed sugars in so many foods) that are fattening.

Some Valuable Suggestions as You Put the Plan into Action

Although the next chapter is loaded with practical tips, I first want to mention a few vital tips as they relate specifically to the eating plan for a day.

Breakfast Tips

If eating only fruit for breakfast just doesn't do it for you, immediately upon waking eat just a little fruit to get your "metabolism motor" started. Try adding some no-fat cottage cheese to some strawberries or other fresh fruit. Use Stevia sweetener if necessary.

Then after getting ready for work, eat as small a breakfast as possible . . . whole-grain cereal (no sugar in the ingredients) with fat-free skim or low-fat milk, fruit on top, and a diet sweetener. Or try Corn Thins with tomato and a half-slice of fat-free cheese melted on top. An omelet, using fat-free cheese, or an egg or two over mashed and heated fat-free refried or pinto beans along with Corn Thins can be eaten. Other ideas include Butter-bean Potato Cakes and Ground-chicken Sausages and Popcorn-flour Pancakes with pureed blueberries or strawberries on top. (See chapter 9 for all recipes.)

On those days when you are famished in the morning, go

ahead and have as much fresh fruit for breakfast as you want. It is imperative that you eat some fruit each and every day—if you don't, you will get terrible cravings for foods with processed sugar—regular sugar—in them and end up going off your diet.

Lunch Tips

You may want to order an extra portion of protein if you are eating out at lunch, or fix an extra portion of protein for yourself. In other words, two chicken breasts instead of one, three burgers instead of two, and so forth. Make sure you are eating sufficient quantities of acceptable soups, salads, and vegetables. Some people simply need more protein to keep from having terrible cravings for snacks in the afternoon, and to help them refrain from eating all the wrong foods at dinnertime.

Make this a positive for you. For example, order or prepare blackened chicken Caesar salad with an extra portion of blackened chicken even as you eliminate the croutons and cheese.

Sometimes you may feel as if you are *forcing* yourself to eat a generous portion of protein at lunch. So be it. Force yourself. The protein will help you stay on your diet.

A valuable note: The longer in the day you can wait to have lunch, the less you will be able to eat for dinner, and the weight will come off even faster.

Snack Tips

Do *not* eat fruit between your daytime meals. If you do, you will eventually get sick of eating fruit and go off your diet. If you get the munchies at night, eat some fresh fruit, fruit salad, raisins, or a fruit smoothie. For snacking between daytime meals, and sometimes at night, see "What About Eating Between Meals," which follows.

The Best Way to Start *Let's Do Lunch*

To begin with, don't worry about losing weight. First, you need to eat *Let's Do Lunch* foods that will eliminate your cravings for the fattening foods that have derailed you in the past. And you need to eat these foods until you are full whenever you are hungry, no matter how often that is and no matter how many calories you consume . . . until your cravings are gone. After that happens, do not eat this way anymore. Instead, follow the *Let's Do Lunch* plan.

Face the Fact that You Are Reversing a Lifelong Habit

For many people, the *Let's Do Lunch* program goes against lifelong habits. But stop to consider why you are eating the way you do. You probably developed bad habits without realizing that you were doing so—either you didn't know you were developing a habit, or you didn't know it was bad. The way the vast majority of people in our society eat every day is just plain "dumb." That doesn't mean *they* are dumb. What they are doing is dumb.

Thanks for sharing your story. I now have stories of my own. I weighed over 400 pounds and have lost over 200 pounds. It's not a diet to me. It's my way of living a full and healthy life! (My wife Peggy lost 50 pounds.) —*B. C., OHIO*

How dumb can we get? We eat our big meal of the day just before going to bed, so all that food just lies there, all night long, in a dormant body, and most of it turns to fat. Think about it: our bodies should be active after eating the big meal of the day, in order to burn all the food we have eaten.

How much dumber can we get? We get up in the morning and try to eat sparingly all day long, so we can pig out at night and get fatter.

The dumbest thing we do? After not eating all night long, trying to eat lightly all day long subjects us to terrible cravings for snacks, and when we snack it almost always is on something fattening. And after eating something fattening, we all feel like we have blown it, so why watch what we eat, at least for the rest of that day?

Think about it logically: When should you eat your big meal of the day? As I've already explained, not at night—and not at breakfast because breakfast food will digest long before the day is through, and you will end up eating a second big meal. You need to be eating your one big protein-rich meal at lunch unless your time prevents it.

Also, remember that FAT-FREE DOES NOT MEAN NON-FATTENING. Regular sugar is fat-free, but I believe it to be totally fattening, and there are lots of fat-free foods with lots of regular sugar in them.

Further, SUGAR-FREE DOES NOT MEAN NONFATTEN-ING. There are lots of sugar-free foods that have very fattening ingredients in them.

Note: To get questions answered and to get new recipes, go to www.letsdolunch.com, click on "message boards" and "Register." To get 71 Laminated Recipe Cards for $15 or to order more books, send a check to "Sunshine" (address herein), or order at our Web site (all proceeds go to charities).

Helpful Tips

And Stark Realities

In this chapter I want to share with you some of the Helpful Tips I picked up along the way. For the most part these are very practical techniques and suggestions—"how to's"—that helped me implement into my everyday life the Big Secrets behind the *Let's Do Lunch* plan. But first, let's face the dreaded Stark Realities. There are only two of them, and the good news is this: the Stark Realities don't need to be discouraging. There's a good side to them.

The Stark Realities Don't Need to Be Discouraging

Stark Reality #1: Fat-free Doesn't Mean Nonfattening.

Foods don't have to have fat grams in them in order to be fattening. For example, processed and refined sugars and syrups have absolutely no fat grams in them—yet they are extremely fattening. In many cases, manufacturers have engineered no-fat and low-fat foods to have *more* sugar in them. The label may not say *sugar,* but the words *glucose, sucrose, syrup,* and *cane juice* mean "sugar." Don't be duped. Read labels, and be wise.

The good side of this Stark Reality is that after you've been on the *Let's Do Lunch* program for two weeks, you won't miss high-fat and high-sugar foods. And, if you *do* have a craving for a fat food, there are ways of meeting that craving without giving in to the most fattening version. Chapter 5 deals with specific cravings. And never forget one of the Big Secrets: choose the least fattening food that tastes good among all the available options. (Instead of sugar in recipes, use Stevia or Splenda sweetener.)

Stark Reality #2: Desserts Are a Thing of the Past.

Perhaps the starkest of the Stark Realities for many people is that desserts are definitely a thing of the past if you are going to lose weight and keep it off. But don't be dismayed because by forcing yourself to eat fruits, especially grapes and frozen grapes, you will actually become addicted to them and you will no longer desire desserts or candy.

If you feel that you must have dessert, try something like strawberries with fat-free cottage cheese and Stevia sweetener sprinkled on, or eat sugar-free Jello, with or without a banana or other fruit in it.

And that's it. Those are the Stark Realities. Let's move ahead to some very common questions people ask about the *Let's Do Lunch* program and some practical tips to help you succeed.

Do You Have Any Suggestions About Eating Fruit?

My wife, Anita, kept a huge fruit salad in a large mixing bowl in the fridge at all times, so that even in the middle of the night I could satisfy my sweet tooth. She made it with a fresh cantaloupe, a honeydew melon, two or three apples, one-and-a-half pounds of green seedless grapes, one and a half pounds of red seedless grapes, two or three oranges, one can of "light" mixed fruits (well drained), and one can of chunky pineapple (also well drained).

She didn't add things like bananas, papayas, mangos, kiwifruit, watermelon, pears, peaches, or strawberries because after sitting they make the fruit salad mushy. If these were added, they were added just before serving.

For breakfast I normally ate only fruit, and I ate as much as I felt like eating. Some days I ate a lot and others not so much. But I almost always tried to eat *some* fruit in order to get enough natural sugar into my system to eliminate later morning cravings and to speed up my metabolism. For some reason I often felt like eating cut-up grapefruit.

When it was time to eat fruit, and I wanted something different, I had a couple of baked apples or apple slices with cinnamon and a little Stevia sweetener sprinkled on them.

Choose Fresh Fruit Whenever Possible.

Eat fresh, frozen, and canned fruits instead of eating applesauce and drinking fruit juices, if possible. Fresh, frozen, and canned fruits will fill you up faster and you'll consume fewer calories.

Enjoy the Benefits of Eating Fruit.

Fruit can have a great benefit—many people, especially older people, find it helpful with their constipation problems. Some people, however, find themselves hurrying to the restroom when they first begin eating a lot of fruit. The body seems to adjust fairly quickly, however, to a new eating habit that includes more fruit, and regularity should be the result for the vast majority of people.

Wash Your Produce Thoroughly.

My wife, Anita, discovered a fruit and veggie wash at the grocery store. She uses it to remove pesticides, sulfates, herbicides, fungicides, and waxes. Eating as much fruit and as many vegetables as we do, we feel safer washing our produce thoroughly.

What Can a Person Do to Satisfy the "Need to Chew"?

When you're not really hungry but you just want to chew on something, put a couple of pieces of diet chewing gum in your mouth and have at it.

What About Eating Between Meals?

Don't eat between meals unless you are extremely hungry. I play golf three times a week with friends, and inevitably at the 19th hole—the clubhouse, for those of you who aren't golfers—many of the guys routinely chow down on burgers and fries. If I'm not extremely hungry, I simply sit and visit while sipping on a glass of tea. If I can't stand to wait until lunchtime or dinnertime, I eat a little something with them, perhaps a bowl of acceptable soup.

Do *not* eat fruit between daytime meals. If you need a snack, you can have one of the following:

- *Carrot sticks* and or other *raw veggies* are nice. You can eat all you want and use a little fat-free or low-fat veggie dip, if necessary.
- *Popcorn.* I like Orville Redenbacher's 94 percent fat-free popcorn. If you don't like it plain, use olive-oil spray, I Can't Believe It's Not Butter spray, or melt a few strips of fat-free cheese over the top in the microwave.
- *Edamame soybeans.* The only ingredients are soybeans and water. These are available in grocery stores or health food stores in several forms. I like them in pod form. You can hold the pod with your teeth and squeeze the beans out. Spray with olive oil, season to taste, and microwave them—they make a wonderful snack that is nonfattening and delicious.

• *Dry-roasted soy nuts.* Be sure these contain no sugar. The ones with sunflower oil or fruit or vegetable oils are okay, and they are delicious. Mix them with raisins and enjoy!

Only if the above options are not acceptable or satisfying to you should you eat the following:

• A couple of Real Foods Original Corn Thins, each with a slice of fat-free cheese melted on top.
• A couple of Corn Thins dipped in salsa or a mixture of mashed and heated fat-free refried beans or pinto beans and a little fat-free cheese

How Often Should a Person Get on the Scales?

When starting *Let's Do Lunch*, it is imperative that you don't weigh yourself for the FIRST month!

When I was dieting and weighing every day, I weighed myself every morning. There were some days I would wake up eight pounds heavier than the day before. To say the least, this was very discouraging. So I decided not to jump on the scale every day. Weighing once a month was perfect for me. If you just can't stand to wait that long, weigh every two weeks. But please don't put yourself through the misery of weighing any more often than once every two weeks, and don't worry about it when your weight plateaus. Keep following the *Let's Do Lunch* program and the weight *will* come off.

What Can I Do if I Get Stuck on a Plateau?

Try my Fruit and Soup Flush (page 65) to jump-start your weight loss again.

Shouldn't a Person Immediately Cut Down on Portion Size?

No. In the beginning of the program, you should not cut down on the amount of food you eat each day.

What Kind of Oil Should a Person Use for Cooking and in Recipes?

Oils are full of fat, except that I believe the oils in fish, soybean oil, and olive oil are nonfattening. I used extra-virgin olive oil nearly all the time, although I occasionally did use corn oil or vegetable oil.

I certainly lost a lot of weight eating vast amounts of salads as main entrees—for example, Caesar salads made with olive oil or soybean oil (including grilled chicken and blackened tuna Caesars), and Italian salads. I especially love the "all you can eat" salad at the Olive Garden restaurants. Of course, I order these salads without cheese and croutons, but with extra tomatoes, onions, and peppers.

How Often Can a Person Eat Red Meat?

I ate red meat often at the beginning of my *Let's Do Lunch* plan. However, I didn't eat it until I got a craving for it. Anita bought the leanest ground beef money could buy, and I ate it until satisfied—with ketchup, sweet relish, tomato, and onion—as the protein for my lunch.

To cut down on my red-meat consumption, I learned to eat other things I liked with it—less fattening or non-fattening things. As I mentioned earlier, I mixed my extra-lean ground beef with ground turkey breast. I also mashed pinto beans and onions into a ground beef and turkey breast mixture, and ate this delicious mixture as "burgers" with the condiments of my choice. It tastes like pure ground beef!

I mixed ground turkey breast with extra-lean ground beef to make chili. I found that the turkey took on the flavor of the beef, so I got the same taste as if I were eating 100 percent beef, but what I was putting into my body was much less fattening.

Likewise, when mashing, blending, or pureeing beans and mixing with beef, you only taste the beef.

Can a Person Have Potatoes, Rice, or Pasta?

My short answer is "almost none."

French fries, American fries, scalloped, twice baked, mashed, au gratin, hash browns, pan fried, potato salad, potato tots, potato pancakes, potato puffs, potato sticks, candied potatoes, and potato chips are out. In fact, a small bag of potato chips can almost equate to eating *all day* on the *Let's Do Lunch* eating program.

For those people who love potatoes, my advice is: don't eat them unless you have an actual craving for them. If you do have a craving, try eating a baked potato with salsa or top it with I Can't Believe It's Not Butter spray or olive oil spray. Avoid using butter, margarine, or sour cream.

If I occasionally just had to have a little pasta, I'd use no-yolk egg noodles and add spaghetti sauce or lots of fresh steamed vegetables with fat-free cheese melted on top. The emphasis was on the toppings, not the pasta.

If you are eating beans, corn, and peas as one of the Big Secrets, you are going to have much less desire for potatoes, rice, or pasta.

If it's rice that you simply must have, eat something with pure wild rice or pure brown rice in it. (See chapter 9 for recipes.)

Can a Person Drink Alcohol on the
Let's Do Lunch Plan?

When I was serious about losing weight as fast as possible, I abstained from alcoholic drinks of any kind. However, after I had lost approximately 190 pounds, I began to drink wine socially again.

It slowed my weight loss, but I continued to lose weight—although as I said, much more slowly—until I had lost an additional forty pounds. For approximately the first year and a half I refrained from drinking, and my weight loss during that time was substantially more each month than it was after I started drinking again. Also, drinking wine caused me to deal with many more cravings than I had when I was abstaining.

Be advised that alcohols from fruits (wine, Ciroc vodka, etc.) are far better for weight loss than other alcohols.

Can a Person Drink Coffee or
Soft Drinks on the Plan?

I didn't drink sugar-loaded soft drinks on my program and I recommend as little diet pop as possible. I didn't lose weight quite as fast when I drank diet pop. I realize that some people are addicted to diet pop, and to them I say, "Drink what you have to because you will still lose the weight." I also encourage them to wean themselves off diet drinks if possible.

My highest recommendation is that a person drink distilled water because it contains no dissolved solids. Anything that is in the body that can dissolve in distilled water will do so and will flush right out of your system. When eating out, I recommend plain old H_2O with a slice of lemon in it, bottled water, or tea. Diet green tea has no calories and is wonderful.

Some coffees, such as cappuccinos or lattes, are very fattening, but plain old brewed or instant flavored coffee—regular or decaf—is okay. However, as was the case with diet pop, I lost weight faster when I drank distilled water, reverse osmosis water, water with a slice of lemon in it, bottled water, or tea. To people who are addicted to coffee, I say drink as little as possible. Also, if you must have cream in your coffee, try to use skim or non-fat milk.

Many diet plans recommend a specific amount of water. I don't. Fruit contains a great deal of water, and most people don't need to drink an additional six to eight glasses of water a day if they are eating sufficient fruit. I do believe, however, that it is a good idea to drink as much water as you like.

Can a Person Have Eggs and Dairy Products?

Let's Do Lunch does include eggs. Some people will want a little skim or nonfat milk in their coffee, and some people will want a little 1 percent or no-fat cottage cheese once in a while. Also, every so often I had low-fat frozen yogurt in a cup—not a cone. Again, eat as little as possible because I believe that even these no-fat or low-fat foods are very fattening.

As I mentioned in telling my story, I love blue cheese. I found that a little blue cheese on a salad could make me want to eat more salad, which was good. I used this cheese sparingly—the sharp taste satisfied me in small quantities—and I still do. Show me a person who eats lots of salads and you'll show me someone who is thin.

The only other cheese I ate was Kraft or Borden fat-free, sharp, processed cheese product. And I only ate this to satisfy my pizza and cheese cravings. Other than this, I abstained from eating cheese. I believe that fat-free cheese *is* fattening—it's just the least fattening form of a fattening food that tastes good to me.

I've been on the *Let's Do Lunch* program for about four months now, and I find it easy to stick to the plan. Last night I tried on all ten pairs of jeans I own to try to find a pair to wear to a party. None of them fit me anymore—they were all too big! I'm down to a size 8 and looking really good. —*S. S., FLORIDA*

Does a Person Take Vitamins or Minerals as Part of this Program?

I recommend that you consult your physician or registered dietitian regarding your vitamin and mineral supplement requirement. It may be wise for you to take a calcium supplement since this program greatly reduces your intake of dairy products.

Are All Fast-Food Items Eliminated in *Let's Do Lunch*?

Fast foods can't be eliminated because of the occasional need for them due to time constraints. Always remember one of the Big Secrets: choose to eat the least fattening food on the menu of all the choices that are appealing. Chapter 6 is about eating out, including eating at fast-food restaurants.

How Do You Keep Diet Food from Being Boring?

I refuse to eat boring food. A person won't stick with any program that eliminates all "taste" from eating. I became a master at using condiments wisely.

For example, I didn't eat corn on the cob "dry." I sprayed a little olive oil on it or used the I Can't Believe It's Not Butter spray. The corn tasted great. I did *not* use actual butter or margarine.

The *Let's Do Lunch* program has lots of acceptable condiments, including barbecue sauce, hot sauce, chili sauce, steak sauce, meatless spaghetti sauce, salsa, vinegar, ketchup, and sweet relish. Check out the shopping list in chapter 8.

When using mayonnaise, I used just enough reduced-fat mayo to hold a tuna salad together and to make my own recipe for tartar sauce. When eating condiments and salad dressings, I always put them on the side. Then, I'd dip my fork into the condiment or dressing just before putting my fork into a bite of food. I ate much less of a condiment or dressing that way, but still had all the benefits of the satisfying taste.

What *Don't* You Eat on the *Let's Do Lunch* Program?

There were lots of foods that I eliminated—but not for the reason you may think. I simply never had a craving for them. Eating fresh fruit took away my great desire for sweets. I found that other substitutions, especially eating corn, peas, and beans, took away my desire for starchy foods. And after a while, things made with a lot of fat or cream tasted too "heavy" to be appealing.

I eliminated the following foods because I just didn't want them any more. I realize this may seem strange to you if you are overweight and struggle to lose weight, but it was true—I lost my desire for the following foods that helped make me fat and kept me fat:

- Appetizers
- Candy
- Chocolate and cocoa
- Creams and creamed foods
- Deep-fried foods
- Fats
- Fruits sweetened or canned in heavy syrup
- Gravies
- Dips

- Guacamole (I still ate avocado on some salads such as a Cobb salad, but in very small quantities—avocadoes have a high fat content.)
- Jam, jelly, and marmalade
- Molasses
- Nuts and seeds (All nuts and seeds are extremely fattening.)
- Processed meats
- Scalloped foods
- Sour cream
- Sugar and sugar products
- Syrups
- Most toppings (such as cheese, cream sauces, gravies)

I *never* ate extremely fattening foods, such as nuts, seeds, and potato chips, because even a small portion of these foods equated to my being able to eat *all day* on the *Let's Do Lunch* program. If you are craving nuts or potato chips, you are usually craving something salty. Try popcorn or dry-roasted soy nuts instead.

I have repeatedly found in talking to people across the nation that once a person has been on the *Let's Do Lunch* program for about two weeks, that person isn't nearly as tempted to eat fattening foods—except on those occasions when the person has had alcohol to drink and his or her mind isn't working properly. Don't allow yourself to get sidetracked by cravings. (Chapter 5 contains suggestions on how to conquer cravings.)

What Happens if I "Fall Off the Wagon" or Eat Fattening Foods?

My advice is to start again on the *Let's Do Lunch* program. It's an easy program to get back on, unlike many diet plans that people just can't bear to restart. I highly recommend my Fruit and Soup Flush as a *must* after a day when you've been bad. Here's what's involved in that flush:

Roger Troy's Fruit and Soup Flush

Eat *nothing* but acceptable fruits, popcorn, or soups that have vegetables, but no potatoes, *for one full day.* Eat as much as you want and as often as you want. Stay away from any soup that has cheese, oil, red meat, potatoes, beer, cream, milk, butter, margarine, gravy, processed meat, or fat of any kind. (See chapter 9 for great soups!)

What About Maintaining the Weight I Lose?

For any eating plan or diet to work for the rest of your life you have to be able to do three things:

1. Eat until you are full.
2. Eat foods you like—without having to eat foods you don't like.
3. Eat whenever you are hungry.

The *Let's Do Lunch* plan is based on these three principles. You also have to be able to satisfy your cravings. *Let's Do Lunch* gives you ways to do that. Eating only foods you love is extremely important because if you don't, your brain eventually will not willingly receive what you are eating, and you will go back to your old fattening ways.

Likewise, if you don't eat until you are satisfied, your brain will know you are still hungry, and sooner or later you'll go back to those old ways.

Satisfying cravings is also crucial, again because *you just can't fool that old brain!* Punishing your brain in this way is like climbing Mt. Everest wearing sneakers—you're going to slip and fall, and then the hurt comes from gaining back more weight than you lost.

I've continued to eat the *Let's Do Lunch* way for more than a decade. The program works. I haven't gained back weight. I don't even think in terms of dieting any longer. This is just the way I eat. And I love it!

Where Did You Get the Name *Let's Do Lunch*?

I realize this isn't exactly a "practical tip," but so many people have asked me this question that I'll answer it here. After I had finished writing the book, I told my wife I was sure that if I looked in the Bible for the passage where Jesus and His disciples fed thousands of people, the name of the book would come to me. So there I was in bed reading through Matthew, Mark, Luke, and John. As I came to the verse where Jesus' disciples were feeding five thousand families with one little boy's lunch, the phone rang. It was my mom, saying, "Honey, I've got the name of the book—*Let's Do Lunch!*" I think you know exactly how I felt at that moment in time—my cup runneth over! I said, "Thank You, Jesus . . . thank you, Mom!"

I truly believe that *Let's Do Lunch* is a gift from God not only to me, but to all mankind. Without this gift I would have died from obesity.

Now we need to pass this gift on to others throughout the world, including our children . . . from the time they are first able to eat regular food and on through their growing-up years. Along this line, we need to get a copy of *Let's Do Lunch* into the hands of our respective school board members, and ask them to change school lunches to *Let's Do Lunch* lunches.

Conquering Cravings

And Avoiding Pitfalls that Are Sure to Arise

Cravings can derail even a strong-willed person. I know. They were what kept me from weight loss for thirty years. I had to develop very specific strategies for conquering those sudden urges to eat foods that I knew were not helpful to my overall goal of losing weight.

Remove as Much Temptation as You Can

The place to start was to throw away all the fattening foods we had in our home. I have to admit, this was hard for me. I don't like to waste money, and I saw lots of money tossed into the trashcan when we started cleaning out our cupboards, refrigerator, and freezer. But it was either "waste" or "on the waist."

Finally I came to realize that throwing away these fattening foods was *not* really a waste at all. This was an investment in my weight loss and my family's health. In discarding old, fattening, unhealthy, harmful foods, I was taking a big step toward living a healthier life.

I encourage you go to chapter 8, and take a quick look through it. This chapter lists the foods that are *acceptable* to have in your home. Make this your inventory list as you clean out your cupboards and pantry.

Get Rid of the Sugar.

First, throw away all the foods you have in your home that have sugar in them, even the fat-free ones. Check the labels on foods. You may be surprised at how many foods have some form of sugar added, although it may be listed as glucose or sucrose. There is a little sugar in some of the sauces and condiments listed in chapter 8, but these are very small amounts in food items that are used sparingly.

Sugar may have no fat grams, but in your body sugar turns to pure fat, and food with sugar in it causes extreme cravings for all the wrong foods.

Throw Away Fattening Leftovers.

As you clear out your pantry and refrigerator, also throw away all leftovers that have fat in them. Especially after throwing a party, it is important to throw away all the fattening foods that have been left over.

Throw Away Coupons and Phone Numbers for Fattening Take-Out.

While you're in the "tossing out" mode, throw away any coupons or phone numbers for fattening take-out foods, especially pizza. A pizza discount coupon can be just as much a temptation as a large pizza in the freezer.

Don't Assume You Can Avoid Cheating.

The hard cold truth is that if you don't have anything fattening around the house, your cravings will rarely get the best of you. Believe me when I say that if you *do* keep fattening, sugary foods around, eventually you will eat them, especially if you have an occasional alcoholic drink, which I have found breaks down will power and creates unbelievable cravings for all the wrong foods.

Confronting What You Are Really Craving

After I had cleared our home of all the wrong foods, I was pretty proud of myself. And then the day came when I had a sudden, unbelievably strong craving for pizza. A *craving* is an uncontrollable lusting for something you've found extremely pleasurable in the past. Believe me, I was *lusting* for pizza on that day!

Fortunately there were no pizzas in the house, and I had no pizza coupons. In the time that it would have taken me to look up the phone number for my favorite pizza delivery service, I sat down and ate a mountain of frozen grapes. That got me through.

Later that night, I realized that what I was really craving was the *cheese* on pizza. I hadn't thought to analyze just which portion of the pizza I was desiring. The good news was that I knew how to satisfy that craving in a less fattening way. I ended up eating a half-slice of fat-free cheese melted on a couple of whole-grain fat-free crispbreads (no sugar).

Another time when that craving for pizza hit me, I ate as much as I wanted of Little Mary's Pizza Soup (see chapter 9). These were the least fattening choices that tasted the best to me. And eating this way worked! I don't remember how much I ate of Pizza Soup at that time, but I know this, my craving was satisfied, and I didn't consume nearly as many calories as in a family-size pizza, which was my usual portion in those days.

My cheese craving was also satisfied in these two ways:

- Real Foods Original Corn Thins, with a slice of tomato and a half-slice of sharp fat-free cheese melted on top.

- Blue cheese crumbles on a salad. These crumbles actually made eating salads more enjoyable for me, and they satisfied my cheese craving at the same time.

I'm skinny for the first time since I was thirteen years old. It's a thrill going from a size 10 to a size 4 in five months.—*M.S., FLORIDA*

When the Craving Was for Bread

As I have stated earlier, I believe that eating bread is like eating a piece of cake, and I loved bread. The truth is, I would rather have had bread than cake.

When a craving for bread hit me, I satisfied this by spreading popcorn out in a large flat dish and spraying it with I Can't Believe It's Not Butter or a 100 percent extra-virgin olive oil spray. Delicious! Or I'd melt a few torn strips of fat-free sharp cheese over the top of the popcorn. Or I'd eat something else with corn, beans, or peas in it. Or I would have a couple of Corn Thins dipped in salsa or a mixture of mashed and heated fat-free refried beans or pinto beans and a little fat-free cheese. My cravings for bread were eventually totally eliminated.

As I related earlier, I also learned a new way to eat a sandwich—open-faced. I've concluded that to eat a sandwich with two slices of bread is to bring on diet failure. A person gets the same taste and satisfaction of bread by eating only one slice.

The best way to eat a sandwich is to have it served on one slice of rye or whole-wheat bread, or to have the sandwich ingredients served on a plate with a whole-grain bun on the side. Cut the bun in half and throw away one half (if you are in a restaurant, put that half in a napkin and set it aside so you can't see it).

Then scoop out the insides of the other half and put the sandwich ingredients in the remaining "hole." You'll still feel as if you've had a full sandwich.

When the Craving Was for Something Sweet

I overcame my craving for sweets by forcing myself to eat fruits whenever I had an urge for pie, cake, ice cream, candy, cookies, or other sugary foods. I admit that this was extremely difficult at first—sugar is highly addictive. But you know what eventually happened? I became addicted to fruit, and I now eat it every day. Especially when I craved the sweet and cold of ice cream, I ate frozen grapes until I was satisfied.

When the Craving Was for Red Meat

I handled my desire for pizza and sweets by making the substitutions I've noted previously, but I faced a real challenge when I had a craving for a thick juicy steak. I just couldn't seem to come up with something that would salve my lifelong craving for red meat. Well, you may have guessed what happened. I had another awakening! This time the concept was that I didn't *have* to find a substitute for red meat. All I had to do was be smarter about eating it.

1. I ate it only when I actually craved it.

2. I chose to eat only the leanest red meat available.

3. I ate meat only at lunch.

4. I ate until I was satisfied—sometimes as much as two pounds of extra-lean ground beef at one meal, each bite eaten

with a fork that had been dipped into on-the-side ketchup, relish, tomato, and onion.

Over time, as my waistline shrank, I had less and less desire for such large quantities of red meat, but I satisfied those cravings in the same way—eating the leanest meat available and only at lunch.

When the Craving Was for Something Salty

My love of salty foods presented yet another challenge. The answer for me? Popcorn or dry-roasted soy nuts! You'll love them.

When I got a salt craving, I thoroughly enjoyed eating a bag of gourmet popping corn, without butter added. For me, the product that tasted the best was Orville Redenbacher's Gourmet Smart-Pop Microwave Popping Corn. That was the least fattening that tasted the best. Would you believe I sometimes happily bloated myself with two bags? I sprayed the popcorn with 100 percent extra-virgin olive oil (Pam brand). I'd love to see the look on your face the first time you try this—you won't believe how good it is!

When my wife, Anita, and I go to an early afternoon movie, we fill up on popcorn—without butter—at the theater. We don't do this often, of course, but we usually find that popcorn at the theater satisfies us for lunch on those days when we are doing *Let's Do Lunch* at dinner.

When the Craving Was for Pasta or Potatoes

Even though I didn't have cravings for pasta or potatoes, Anita did. She found that those cravings were solved when she ate something with corn, beans, or peas in it. (See chapter 9.)

And What About the Times When I Didn't Know What I Wanted?

Most of the time, I found that I could avoid eating something very fattening by choosing something else on my program that also appealed to me. At times, however, I found myself wanting something really substantial, but not knowing what it was. When that happened I'd simply go through my Ultimate Grocery Shopping List (chapter 8) until something struck my fancy. If nothing appealed to me, I would look for something on my list of foods "to go" (see The Best Take-Out Food on pages 85–86).

Cravings Can Be Intense After Drinking Alcohol

Let me warn you that cravings seem to be especially intense after drinking alcohol. After I started drinking a little wine again—and keep in mind, I'd already lost 190 pounds at that point—I found that on the rare occasions when I drank too much wine, I had some of the most difficult cravings I'd ever dealt with. I'd have an almost uncontrollable urge for all the foods I knew I should not consume.

I especially wanted pizza in the worst way. When that happened, I usually bargained with myself that if I filled up on fruit first—even though I definitely didn't want any—and then waited for a half hour, I could have a pizza. I found that when the time came to eat the pizza, I was able to control the amount that I ate because of the vast amount of natural fruit sugar already in my system. If I didn't eat the fruit, I couldn't seem to stop eating the pizza.

Finally, I figured out a way to get by without eating any pizza. If I was still hungry after eating fruit, I forced myself to eat soup until my stomach looked like a balloon that had just been filled with water. Or I bloated myself with popcorn sprayed with olive oil or topped with little strips of fat-free cheese. Occasionally, I'd eat a couple of crispbreads, each with a tomato slice and a half-slice of fat-free cheese melted on top.

To avoid drinking too much wine, Anita drinks a glass of water between each glass. I think that's a super idea for any person who chooses to drink.

Several Questions About Cravings

I have repeatedly been asked the following questions about cravings:

Question: How do I overcome my craving for a Coke in the morning?

Answer: First of all, you are probably really craving either caffeine or refined sugar. If it's refined sugar, be sure to eat fruits every day—especially the sweetest ones like raisins, grapes, pineapple, and watermelon. If it's caffeine, try drinking tea or coffee, but as little as possible. It this doesn't work, try getting rid of your caffeine and sugar addictions with the following approach:

For one week, drink ¾ Coke and ¼ diet Coke in a large glass filled with lots of ice. The next week, drink half regular Coke and half diet Coke. The third week, drink ¼ Coke with ¾ diet Coke, and then drink straight diet Coke. Next, take on your caffeine addiction the same way. Drink ¾ regular diet Coke and ¼ decaffeinated diet Coke for one week. The next week move to a half-and-half combination. The third week drink ¼ caffeinated and ¾ decaffeinated diet Coke. And finally, drink only decaffeinated diet Coke for a week. After that, switch to water, and drink plenty of it.

A friend of mine followed this method for getting rid of a caffeine and sugar addiction, and it really worked. If you go cold turkey after developing a regular habit of lots of caffeine and sugar in a day, you'll likely get headaches or feel sick, which means you'll get discouraged and give up trying. A gradual method works much better and is doable for the vast majority of people.

Question: How do I overcome my craving for a sub sandwich every day?

Answer: You are probably craving bread. Read my suggestions about that earlier in this chapter. If nothing works, go for it, but throw half the bun away, and be sure to have a sandwich that doesn't contain processed meats. Stick with meats you can lose weight with—skinless chicken and skinless turkey breast.

Question: How do I keep from craving the cookies I love so much?

Answer: You are probably craving refined sugar. Start eating a lot of raisins, grapes, pineapple, and watermelon in order to get fructose (fruit sugar) into your system. Over time, you will likely start craving fruit instead of cookies!

Question: I love peanut butter and nuts. What can I do about this?

Answer: You are probably craving protein. When this craving strikes, you need to eat the leanest red meat available, and as much as is necessary to satisfy your craving. I recommend extra-lean ground sirloin with your favorite condiments on the side.

Dry roasted soy nuts are a great snack to satisfy a craving for nuts. Just be sure they have no coatings. If necessary, spray them with a bit of olive oil and a little salt and heat in the oven or microwave.

Question: If I'm at a party and I'm craving the brownies or other sweets that are served, what do I do?

Answer: Anticipate this in advance. Have some fruit before you go to the party. Force yourself to eat some sweet fruit every day. This will keep the craving for sugary foods from building up.

Question: What if nothing I try satisfies the craving for a particular food?

Answer: If you just can't eliminate a craving for a certain food, then eat as little as possible and as seldom as possible—and choose the least fattening version of the food.

Anticipating and Avoiding Pitfalls

Even though the *Let's Do Lunch* program addresses all the major obstacles involved with losing weight, there are four pitfalls to avoid and guard against:

1. If you don't eat fruit every day, you could develop terrible cravings for sweets that could force you off the program.

You may have to force yourself to eat fruits over a short period of time, but eventually, you'll find yourself absolutely not enticed by things such as family-size chocolate bars, cookies, cakes, éclairs, and all the other foods made with processed and refined sugar. When I was 425 pounds, if you put a chocolate bar anywhere within one hundred yards of me it would be gone before the wrapper had a chance to settle on the table. After I began this program and was on it for a few weeks, I wasn't the least bit interested in candy.

If you eat large quantities of foods—fat free or not—with substantial amounts of processed and refined sugars or syrups in them, you will likely experience the following consequences:

- Your weight loss will be slowed or stopped because processed sugars and syrups are very fattening even though they contain no fat grams.
- You will feel hungrier, with the desire to eat only fattening foods.
- You may want to eat continuously.
- You could have irresistible urges (cravings) for more fattening foods that have processed sugars and syrups in them.
- You are likely to become easily irritable.
- You may feel very tired.

I am a 79-year-old male, retired family physician. I read about "Let's Do Lunch" in September 2003 in the Jackson, MS *Clarion-Ledger*. . . I lost a total of 20 pounds (from 228 to 208) in 8 weeks. I have continued to use the principles of the diet to maintain my weight between 205 and 210. I highly recommend this program to anyone unless contraindicated by their own personal physician. —*R. L. B., MISSISSIPPI*

2. Anticipate the alcohol questions and temptations in advance.

Drinking buddies often aren't the least bit sympathetic to your weight loss program, and they are likely to continue to offer you the same kind of fattening drinks you used to partake of. In my case, someone was always buying me a brandy Manhattan without my asking for it.

If you have decided that on the *Let's Do Lunch* program you are not going to drink, then simply pull the bartender or server aside and tell him that you are going to be ordering screwdrivers (or Bloody Marys), but that you want plain orange juice or tomato juice delivered to your table instead.

If, on the other hand, you have decided that on the *Let's Do Lunch* program you *are* going to drink—thus losing weight more slowly—then simply tell your buddies that you have become a wine drinker, and order only a glass of wine. Remember that drinking brings on extreme cravings and will sabotage your will power.

3. Anticipate what you will tell a host.

If you are going to a party or are visiting a friend or relative overnight, stop at a local grocery store on the way and buy fruit. Tell your host you are on a health program in which you must eat some fruit, and then eat any other foods offered to you according to the *Let's Do Lunch* program. If you are going to a dinner party, plan in advance to make that one of the days in which you do the *Let's Do Lunch* program for dinner (having your protein at night)—again, eat according to the program. Be sure to buy enough fruit so you can share with your host and any other guests.

4. Anticipate your role as a host.

If your guests have their hearts set on eating fried chicken, then fix the fried chicken for them, and fix your chicken according to the *Let's Do Lunch* way. You'll both be eating chicken, but with one difference—you will continue to lose weight!

Eating Out

And Safely Navigating the Fast-Food
Drive-Through

As is true for many people trying to lose weight, I faced a challenge when it came to eating out. I had to learn that when I was on the road it was possible to safely navigate fast-food drive-through lanes at places such as McDonald's. Following are some of my eating-out strategies:

I Ordered Food "My Way"

At a restaurant, I ordered food the way I wanted it—not the way it was presented on the menu. For example, instead of pecan crusted fish, I ordered blackened or grilled fish.

Just as I prepared foods at home, I ordered my nonfattening food in a way that I'd enjoy it—in other words, adding the least fattening thing possible that made the taste likable—and yes, I still lost weight! In the case of ordering blackened or grilled fish, I also ordered tartar sauce on the side. I dipped my fork into the tartar sauce before taking each bite of fish. It worked just as well in a restaurant as at my own kitchen table.

At times, I asked my wife to help me by bringing along a

couple of Corn Thins and a container of my own recipe for tartar sauce (see chapter 9). Her purse is large enough to hide these items! The Corn Thins were just in case I got an urge for a dinner roll.

As another example, I found that nearly all restaurants are prepared to make an omelet, and usually one with egg substitute. I ordered an Egg Beaters omelet *without* cheese but with tomatoes, onions, green peppers, and salsa. I asked that green beans and corn replace anything else that was normally served with an omelet at no extra charge. I found that restaurants happily made this adjustment.

If I found myself at a place where an Egg Beaters omelet was not available—such as a Perkins or a Cracker Barrel restaurant—I ordered a regular omelet without cheese but with veggies in the middle and tomatoes on the side, and I ate salsa on the top. Or I ordered scrambled eggs and asked that they prepare them in a pan with olive oil. If they made a mistake and fried them in butter, I would discreetly blot them with a napkin.

I Adjusted Foods as They Came to the Table

Sometimes it's just not possible to order things "your way," but you can usually remove some ingredients from dishes to make them conform to your plan. For example, at Chinese restaurants I felt fine about ordering moo goo gai pan (a chicken dish) or chicken chow mein but not anything "sub gum" because it had nuts in it. As I shared previously, I always say "nuts" to nuts because the fat goes right to the thighs and the stomach. I found that I liked cashew chicken, however, better than either moo goo gai pan or chicken chow mein—it tasted better to me—and I had no problem removing the cashews when the dish arrived at the table.

I Created New Menu Items

I was never afraid to ask for something that wasn't on the menu. For example, I often ordered a veggie plate that had corn, peas, green beans, lima beans, pinto beans, cole slaw, cooked carrots, or other items. Usually I requested four or five items.

I Became an Expert at Turning Fattening Dishes into Not-So-Fattening Ones

If nonfattening foods on the menu were just not tempting, then I chose something fattening that I could turn into something not so fattening. For example, I ordered:

- Fried chicken, and then I removed the fried skin.
- Eggplant parmigiana or veal parmigiana, and I removed the cheese on top, eating only the red sauce.
- Cobb salad, without croutons and bacon, but with a dressing of my choice served on the side. I love the blue cheese that traditionally comes with this salad, but I took most of that off, leaving only a little. I dipped my fork in the dressing and took a bite of the salad.

Many times I brought my own reduced-calorie dressing to a restaurant—again, relying on Anita's purse as the carrier of my contraband. I personally found that the "least fattening dressings that taste the best" are Newman's Own Dressings. These dressings come in individual packets. Anita goes to McDonald's and buys a dozen or so at a time, and then refrigerates them. Each packet contains enough dressing for two salads. If you don't bring along your own dressing, don't worry—just order your choice on the side.

- A tuna salad sandwich, but served open-face, on just one slice of rye bread.
- Eggs, with salsa on the side. If the eggs looked greasy, I discreetly took several clean napkins and blotted off as much grease as possible.
- An Italian salad, but I asked the server *not* to bring the bread sticks and to leave the cheese and croutons off the salad, replacing them with additional tomatoes, hot peppers, and onions.
- A Caesar salad, with blackened tuna or grilled chicken, but without cheese or croutons.

I Made Smart Choices at Salad Bars

At any food establishment with a salad bar—regular restaurant, fast-food chain, or grocery store—I loaded up my greens with tomatoes, green peppers, onions, beets, and a three-bean salad (all nonfattening), and then I chose a diet dressing. If I had to choose a fattening dressing because I didn't like any of the diet ones, I'd put it on the side and dip my fork in it before each bite.

I am a senior citizen who has tried to eat healthy my entire adult life . . . I have never felt the need to diet and have not followed a diet program . . . that is until I read *Let's Do Lunch.*

Your premise that the *Let's Do Lunch* program will leave its followers with no food cravings intrigued me . . . The cravings I hoped to eliminate were for ice cream and bread and butter. Two weeks after following the program, my unhealthy cravings were gone, and to my surprise I lost 10 pounds. Needless to say, I am hooked on *Let's Do Lunch* and will be eating this way for the rest of my life. —N. M., *INDIANA*

You *Can* Survive Fast-Food Meals

I made it something of a game to see how I might turn a fast-food meal into one that was less fattening. Here are a few of the things I ordered at fast-food establishments:

At Taco Bell and Other Fast-Food Mexican Restaurants

I ordered a chicken taco salad, without avocado, sour cream, guacamole, and cheese—in other words, without the toppings—but with a side order of refried beans, if beans weren't in the salad. Then I'd eat everything but the shell. Yes, I did eat the salsa, or the mild and hot sauces that were available. If one taco salad prepared this way was not enough, I'd order two. To this day I sometimes order two salads like this and scarf them down with sensuous pleasure, leaving the shells on the plate.

At McDonald's and Similar Hamburger Establishments

I ordered a hamburger, threw away the bottom half of the bun, and then took a clean napkin and blotted as much grease off the meat as possible.

I ordered a salad, with a Newman's Own Dressing—I sometimes ordered this for breakfast. Try it—you might like it too!

If I ordered a McGrilled chicken sandwich, I ordered it without cheese and with their sauce on the side. Then I threw away the bottom half of the bun and spread on only a light layer of the sauce.

I ordered scrambled eggs—again blotting off any excess grease—and an apple bran muffin but with *no* butter.

When I only wanted a little something, I ordered a low-fat frozen yogurt cone, put it upside down in a cup, and ate everything but the fattening cone itself.

At Kentucky Fried Chicken and Other Primarily Chicken Establishments

I ordered white meat chicken and corn on the cob. I removed the fried skin and blotted off the oil on the chicken and the butter on the corn.

Surviving Shopping: Trips and Snack Attacks

Eating in a less fattening way at restaurants and fast-food establishments started when I was on my fast track of weight loss. But now, that way of eating is routine for me. It has become a habit.

In my fat days I hardly ever thought twice about how much grease might be on a food or on the plate surrounding it. Now, I'm very aware of it. In the past I didn't think about how much of my food was smothered in cheese and heavy cream sauces. Now, I'm sensitive to that, and I find that the cheese and cream sauces just don't appeal to me anymore. I wouldn't have thought that possible when I was overweight, but now it's true!

Eating out for breakfast, lunch, and dinner weren't my only battle zones, of course. Whenever I went shopping, ran errands, or was traveling, I almost always got the munchies. To solve this problem, I took along some grapes, raisins, or a bag of popcorn or dry-roasted soy nuts.

My wife had her own strategy for addressing the munchies. She'd put raisins, grapes, or a sectioned grapefruit into a plastic bag and eat this fruit in between shopping errands so she wasn't tempted to stop and buy chocolate candy. She found that right before and during her menstrual period, both raisins and grapes quelled her craving for sweets like nothing else could.

Surviving a Party the *Let's Do Lunch* Way

There's good dieting advice that's been around for decades: if you are going to a party, eat before you go. You'll be much better able to resist the temptation of foods that you know are fattening. Be sure to eat fruit so you'll be able to withstand the temptation of sugary or sweet foods and desserts.

Have an answer prepared for a host or hostess. I like these:

- "I had a very late lunch."
- "That looks delicious, and perhaps I'll have some later." In your mind, add these words: like five years from now.
- "No, thank you—not right now." A simple "no, thank you" often is the most direct answer. Say it with a smile.

Cocktails, anyone? Although I am not an every-day drinker, I did find myself with the urge to imbibe every once in a while when I was at a party. However, because I believe drinking severely inhibits weight loss, I basically abstained during my weight-loss time. Let me remind you that my last forty pounds came off much more slowly because I had added a little wine to my diet. I believe those pounds would have been much quicker to lose if I had continued to abstain from all alcohol. Let me also add that I believe drinking grain alcohol slows down weight loss even more than grape alcohol. Grains are fattening in all forms. Grain alcohols include beer and many hard liquors.

The Best Take-Out Food

All of the restaurant and fast-food suggestions offered earlier in this chapter are good for times when you need to stop and pick up something to take home to eat. As I was losing weight, I also enjoyed these foods:

- I'd stop by the Olive Garden and take home an order of eggplant or veal parmigiana. Before heating it up at home, I'd discard the cheese.
- Grocery stores that have salad bars are great for making a salad for one or two on the way home. Be sure to choose the right items for your salad. I like one with sliced tomatoes, green peppers, onions, peas, pickled beets, and three-bean salad.
- Grocery stores often have barbecued or roasted chickens. Some also have roasted turkey breasts that are fully cooked, hot, and ready to go. Be sure to remove the skin from the chicken or turkey.
- I often stopped by a deli to get already-prepared three-bean salad. It was made with oil, but I drained off the oil as soon as I got home.
- It was easy for me to stop and pick up chicken chow mein, plain chow mein, or moo goo gai pan. I threw away the rice and noodles, both crisp and regular, or asked the restaurant just to give me items without rice and noodles.

Sometimes "Eating Out" Is Eating at Your Workplace

The *Let's Do Lunch* recipes certainly can be made in advance and taken on a brown bag basis to work. I recommend that you fix the recipe after you have had a smoothie in the evening so you will not be tempted by the protein in the recipes that are geared for lunch. You can also take the basic ingredients with you to work and concoct your recipe on site, especially if your workplace has a microwave in the kitchen.

Some people find that it's helpful to eat lunch at their desks, rather than go to a cafeteria or be around people who are eating fattening foods. Others don't mind at all eating with others and find the social interaction helpful. They just enjoy their own food as if they were eating out at a restaurant while following the *Let's Do Lunch* program. Here are some additional tips that can help:

1. Be sure to have enough fruit available to you at work so you can fill up on it in case you have a sudden craving for something really fattening. You can do this in several ways.

- Carry a cooler to work. Fill it with fruits you like and enough ice packs to keep them cold.
- Put a small refrigerator in your place of business to hold the fruits you like. If that's not possible, take fruits such as grapes, apples, and grapefruit to work. These fruits can sit out all day and not spoil.
- Take pop-top cans of fruit—ones that have been packed only in their own fruit juices—and drain them before eating.

2. If your workplace does not have a small microwave oven or a small electric two-sided grill, buy these appliances and put them in your workplace kitchen. That way you can make popcorn at work and also grill proteins for lunch.

3. Don't be bashful about sharing *Let's Do Lunch* with other people. Someone may decide to join you on the program. It's always more fun and encouraging if you have a buddy with whom to prepare and eat lunch.

4. Many people find it helpful to eat and then do something else during the lunch hour. One person I know took her lunch to

a park in the spring and summer, and enjoyed the five-block walk to and from the park. Another person drove to a golf driving range a half mile from work, and after eating lunch, which took about fifteen minutes, he had twenty minutes a day to hit golf balls. Yet another person told me that he worked next to a YMCA, and at noon three days a week, he went to the Y to swim for a half hour, then came back and ate lunch. He managed to work it all into an hour.

This brings up the possibility of exercise, of course. I promised you at the outset of this book, and I hold to that promise, that you do *not* need to exercise to lose weight on the *Let's Do Lunch* plan. Let me also say:

- If you are more active, you will likely lose weight a little faster.
- If you do specific weight-bearing exercises a few times a week, you are likely to have a more toned body. As you lose weight, you'll feel and look even better.
- As you lose weight, you are likely to have more energy and a greater desire to be more active. My wife played tennis and walked while she was on the program, not because she felt like she had to, but because she truly enjoys playing tennis and walking.
- Active doesn't mean exercise. Gardening is an activity that a great number of people enjoy. Gardening has a lot of motion in it, and perhaps even some weight lifting, yet hardly anybody thinks of gardening as exercise.

My foremost recommendation about exercise and activity is that you do what is fun for you. Do what you like to do when it comes to activity. The more you engage in that activity, the more satisfied you will be as a human being.

Let me also say this to those people who tell me that they

exercise regularly and just can't seem to lose any weight no matter how active they are or how many miles they log on a treadmill or exercise bike: the truth is, you are probably eating rolls, bread, pasta, crackers, potatoes, fat-free foods with sugar, and other fattening foods—and often are adding butter and margarine to them. There's no way you can work your buns off exercising and then eat buns at noon and night and lose weight.

Right before I started the *Let's Do Lunch* program, I was exercising at least one and a half hours a day—that's right, ninety minutes! I gained forty-five pounds while I was exercising that much. It took me three months to lose those forty-five pounds after I started the *Let's Do Lunch* program. And I lost those pounds by eating right and *not* exercising. I did play golf, using a golf cart.

A friend knew how desperate I was to lose weight. I am a retired body builder and a former beauty pageant winner, but I've also had a clogged artery and mild heart attack. Since I've been on heart medication, I gained weight. I turned into a person I didn't know—with 30 extra pounds on my body I felt like a rock. I did everything I knew to do to lose weight, and I did manage to lose a few pounds, but it took me almost two years of struggling and starving and exercising. Then I was told about your program. In the first 2 weeks I lost 9 pounds. I wasn't hungry once, and I can't tell you how good I feel. I'm on my way! I just had my yearly blood work done and all is good. The doctor asked me what I had been doing differently, and I said, "Let's Do Lunch!" —S. S., FLORIDA

If you crave rice, eat as little as possible of dark rice with the husks still attached. If you crave potatoes, eat as little as possible of a sweet potato.

Every day when it's possible, eat a large portion of foods that make you feel less hungry—like recipes with all the different beans in them, including bean soups. (Remember, you can't taste the beans in most of the recipes . . . for example, Tomato Soup, Pizza Soup, Beef Potato Pie, Tamale Pie, and *Let's Do Lunch* Burgers)

People are always asking me what to eat for breakfast. Except for fruits and fruit smoothies, eat as little as possible and choose from the following: Corn Thins with fat-free cheese, whole-grain cereal (no sugar) with fruit on top, mashed and heated fat-free refried beans with eggs on top, Butter-bean Potato Cakes, Ground-chicken Sausages, and Popcorn-flour Pancakes with pureed blueberries or strawberries on top (see chapter 9).

To insure you get the leanest meat, buy a hand grinder or a Kitchen Aid with grinder attachment.

If you find yourself running to the restroom all the time, you can purchase a product called Imodium that should take care of that problem (get your doctor's approval).

If you find yourself with constipation, eat fresh fruits, drink fruit smoothies, or purchase a product called Metamucil.

Once your sweet cravings are gone, you should not be eating fruits and fruit smoothies except at breakfast, at dinner, and in between dinner and breakfast the next morning. If you eat them more often than this, you will not want them when you should be eating them.

A few ingredients listed in recipes herein are only being used because of no other choice.

Note: If you can't find a particular Let's Do Lunch *food at your local grocery store, then you should be able to find it at a health food store or online.*

7

14-Day Meal Guide

For Those Who Like a Little More Structure

L*et's Do Lunch* is not a structured or regimented program. It is not a breakfast, snack, lunch, snack, dinner, snack plan. You are not required to eat specific portions of specific foods at specific times, which is one of the reasons *Let's Do Lunch* works for everyone.

The following is for those folks who *like* structure and regimentation. As one woman said to me, "The only decision I want to make for a little while is a decision to do the *Let's Do Lunch* program. I want everything else laid out for me." Okay. Here it is—two weeks worth of a predetermined plan!

You can find all the recipes mentioned here in chapter 9. The recipes are sorted by type of food—for example, beef—and then alphabetically by the recipe name.

Remember, if you are not hungry at mealtime, it is not necessary for you to eat!

Day 1

▲ **Breakfast** *(Eat as much as you want.)*
—A banana and all the fresh fruit you want or fruit smoothies. You may want to add no-fat cottage cheese to your strawberries or other fresh fruit. If you must sweeten the fruit to make it enjoyable, use Stevia sweetener. If you just don't feel like fruit, try a glass of V8 juice and a couple of Wasa Light Crispbread or Corn Thins with fat-free cheese melted on top. Or try a little fat-free yogurt.

● **Let's Do Lunch** *(Eat as much as you want.)*
—Neet's Meatloaf with condiments of choice (chapter 9)
—Danita's Three-Bean Salad Delight (chapter 9)
—Bill's Mashed Potatoes (chapter 9)

■ **Dinner** *(Eat as much as you want, but no protein entrée.)*
—A banana and fruit smoothies or fresh fruit
—Then, *if still hungry*: Jimbro and Leelu's Tomato Soup with popcorn on top (chapter 9), and salad of choice with dressing of choice

▼ **Evening snack,** *if still hungry*
—Frozen, seedless grapes and raisins, or popcorn, or dry roasted soy nuts

Day 2

▲ **Breakfast** *(Eat as much as you want.)*
—A banana and all the fresh fruit you want or fruit smoothies, followed by *one* of the following:

- One or two eggs over mashed and heated fat-free refried beans or pinto beans with a couple of Corn Thins
- Popcorn with olive oil sprayed on top (or I Can't Believe It's Not Butter)
- Veggie omelet with fat-free cheese
- Butter-bean Potato Cakes (see chapter 9)

Switch the regular Let's Do Lunch plan to dinner on this day.

▇ **Lunch** *(Eat as much as you want,* but no protein entrée and no fruit.*)*
—Eddie's Hearty Homemade Vegetable Soup (chapter 9)
—Salad of choice with a few blue cheese crumbles and dressing of choice
—Veggies of choice

● **Let's Do Lunch** at Dinner *(Eat as much as you want.)*
—A banana and fruit smoothies or fresh fruit, followed by:

- Salad of choice with dressing of choice
- Ty's Beef and Beans (chapter 9) with Danita's Salsa (chapter 9), or with condiments of choice
- Bill's Mashed Potatoes (chapter 9)

Day 3

▲ **Breakfast** *(Eat as much as you want.)*
—A banana and all the fresh fruit you want or fruit smooth-
ies or V8 juice and a couple of Wasa Light Crispbread or
Corn Thins with fat-free cheese melted on top.

● **Let's Do Lunch** *(Eat as much as you want.)*
—Fred's Caesar Salad (chapter 9)
—Veggies of choice
—Jerry's Easy Beef Stew (chapter 9)
—Bill's Mashed Potatoes (chapter 9)

■ **Dinner** *(Eat as much as you want,* but no protein entrée.)
—A banana and fruit smoothies or fresh fruit
—Then, *if still hungry:* Loerita's Quick Bean Soup (chapter 9)

▼ **Evening snack,** *if still hungry*
—Popcorn with olive-oil spray or I Can't Believe It's Not
Butter

Day 4

▲ **Breakfast** *(Eat as much as you want.)*
—A banana and all the fresh fruit you want or fruit smoothies or V8 juice and a couple of Wasa Light Crispbread with fat-free cheese melted on top.

● **Let's Do Lunch** *(Eat as much as you want.)*
—Salad of choice with a few blue cheese crumbles and dressing of choice
—Veggies of choice
—Gayle's Chicken with Cranberries and Oranges (chapter 9)

■ **Dinner** *(Eat as much as you want, but no protein entrée.)*
—A banana and fruit smoothies or fresh fruit
—Then, *if still hungry:* tomato soup with popcorn on top

▼ **Evening snack,** *if still hungry*
—Sugar-free Jell-O with assorted fruit in it, topped with a little Cool Whip Lite

Day 5

▲ **Breakfast** *(Eat as much as you want.)*
—A banana and all the fresh fruit you want or fruit smoothies, followed by *one* of the following:

• One or two eggs over mashed and heated fat-free refried beans or pinto beans with a couple of Corn Thins
• Popcorn with olive oil sprayed on top (or I Can't Believe It's Not Butter)
• Veggie omelet with fat-free cheese
• Butter-bean Potato Cakes (see chapter 9)

Switch Let's Do Lunch to dinner on this day.

▪ **Lunch** *(Eat as much as you want,* but no protein entrée and no fruit.)
—Vegetable soup (no potatoes, pasta, or rice)
—Salad of choice with a few blue cheese crumbles and dressing of choice
—Veggies of choice

● **Let's Do Lunch** at Dinner *(Eat as much as you want.)*
—A banana and fruit smoothies or fresh fruit, followed by:

• Salad of choice with dressing of choice
• Veggies of choice
• Ron's Awesome Chili (chapter 9)
• Bill's Mashed Potatoes (chapter 9)

Day 6

▲ *Breakfast (Eat as much as you want.)*
—A banana and all the fresh fruit you want or fruit smoothies. Try adding no-fat cottage cheese with your strawberries or other fresh fruit. Sweeten with Stevia sweetener. If
fruit doesn't do it for you, try V8 juice and a couple of
Corn Thins with tomato slice and a half-slice of fat-free
cheese melted on top.

● *Let's Do Lunch (Eat as much as you want.)*
—Salad of choice with dressing of choice
—Veggies of choice
—Del's Grilled Tuna with Ty's tartar sauce (chapter 9)
—Bill's Mashed Potatoes (chapter 9)

■ *Dinner (Eat as much as you want,* but no protein entrée.)
—A banana and fruit smoothies or fresh fruit
—Then, *if still hungry:* Suzie's Spicy Black Bean Soup
(chapter 9)

▼ *Evening snack, only if hungry*
—Veggies with Mattie Lou's Curry Dip (chapter 9)

Day 7

▲ **Breakfast** *(Eat as much as you want.)*
—A banana and all the fresh fruit you want or fruit smoothies or V8 juice and a couple of Wasa Light Crispbread or Corn Thins with fat-free cheese melted on top.

● **Let's Do Lunch** *(Eat as much as you want.)*
—Salad of choice with a few blue cheese crumbles and dressing of choice
—Veggies of choice
—Bob's Key Lime Chicken (chapter 9)

▪ **Dinner** *(Eat as much as you want, but no protein entrée.)*
—A banana and fruit smoothies or fresh fruit
—Then, *if still hungry:* Joanie's Minestrone Soup (chapter 9)

▼ **Evening snack,** *if still hungry*
—Edamame pods sprayed with olive oil, seasoned, and microwaved. Hold the stem end of the edamame pod, and pull it through your teeth, eating only the beans that pop out.

I had a goal of losing 30 pounds. I've lost 36! I was a size 18, and now I'm a size 12. I am not that young anymore so a size 12 is just fine! —G. D., *MAINE*

Day 8

▲ **Breakfast** *(Eat as much as you want.)*
—A banana and all the fresh fruit you want or fruit smoothies or V8 juice and a couple of Wasa Light Crispbread with fat-free cheese melted on top.

● **Let's Do Lunch** *(Eat as much as you want.)*
—Salad of choice with dressing of choice
—Bill's Bean Cakes (chapter 9)
—R.M.'s Made Rights (chapter 9)
—Bill's Mashed Potatoes (chapter 9)

▦ **Dinner** *(Eat as much as you want,* but no protein entrée.)
—A banana and fruit smoothies or fresh fruit
—Then, *if still hungry:* Danita's Salsa (chapter 9) over pinto beans

▼ **Evening snack,** *if still hungry*
—Ange's Crunchy Waldorf Salad (chapter 9)

Day 9

▲ **Breakfast** *(Eat as much as you want.)*
—A banana and all the fresh fruit you want or fruit smoothies, followed by *one* of the following:

- One or two eggs over mashed and heated fat-free refried beans or pinto beans with a couple of Corn Thins
- Popcorn with olive oil sprayed on top (or I Can't Believe It's Not Butter)
- Veggie omelet with fat-free cheese
- Butter-bean Potato Cakes (see chapter 9)

Switch Let's Do Lunch to dinner on this day.

■ **Lunch** *(Eat as much as you want,* but no protein entrée and no fruit.)
—Joel Lynn's Seven Layer Salad (chapter 9)
—Jimbro and Leelu's Mushroom Soup (chapter 9)
—Veggies of choice

● **Let's Do Lunch** at Dinner *(Eat as much as you want.)*
—A banana and fruit smoothies or fresh fruit, followed by:

- Soup of choice
- Tyra's Taco Salad (chapter 9)
- Bill's Mashed Potatoes (chapter 9)

Day 10

▲ **Breakfast** *(Eat as much as you want.)*
—A banana and all the fresh fruit you want or fruit smoothies. Try adding no-fat cottage cheese with your strawberries or other fresh fruit. Sweeten with Stevia. If fruit doesn't
do it for you, try V8 juice with no-fat cottage cheese. Or try
a little fat-free yogurt.

● **Let's Do Lunch** *(Eat as much as you want.)*
—Salad of choice with a few blue cheese crumbles and dress-
ing of choice
—Veggies of choice
—Nancy's Tuna Roll (chapter 9)
—Bill's Mashed Potatoes (chapter 9)

■ **Dinner** *(Eat as much as you want,* but no protein entrée.*)*
—A banana and fruit smoothies or fresh fruit
—Then, *if still hungry:* Bill's Bean Cakes with salsa (chapter 9)

▼ **Evening snack,** *if still hungry*
—Dry-roasted soy nuts sprayed with olive oil, seasoned, and
microwaved

Day 11

▲ **Breakfast** *(Eat as much as you want.)*
—A banana and all the fresh fruit you want or fruit smoothies or V8 juice and a couple of Corn Thins with tomato
slice and fat-free cheese melted on top.

● **Let's Do Lunch** *(Eat as much as you want.)*
—Salad of choice with a few blue cheese crumbles and dress-
ing of choice
—Veggies of choice
—Charlie's Blackened Fish with Ty's Tartar Sauce (chapter 9)
—Bill's Mashed Potatoes (chapter 9)

▦ **Dinner** *(Eat as much as you want,* but no protein entrée.)
—A banana and fruit smoothies or fresh fruit
—Then, *if still hungry:* Pat's Quick Coleslaw and Beans
(chapter 9)

▼ **Evening snack,** *if still hungry*
—Ange's Crunchy Waldorf Salad (chapter 9)

Day 12

▲ *Breakfast (Eat as much as you want.)*
—A banana and all the fresh fruit you want or fruit smoothies, followed by *one* of the following:

- One or two eggs over mashed and heated fat-free refried beans or pinto beans with a couple of Corn Thins
- Popcorn with olive oil sprayed on top (or I Can't Believe It's Not Butter)
- Veggie omelet with fat-free cheese
- Butter-bean Potato Cakes (see chapter 9)

Switch Let's Do Lunch to dinner on this day.

■ *Lunch (Eat as much as you want, but no protein entrée and no fruit.)*
—Martha's Broccoli Cauliflower Salad (chapter 9)
—Tomato soup with mixed veggies added (no potatoes, pasta, or rice)

● *Let's Do Lunch* at Dinner *(Eat as much as you want.)*
—A banana and fruit smoothies or fresh fruit, followed by:

- Salad of choice with dressing of choice
- Veggies of choice
- Tyra's Chicken Parmesan (chapter 9)
- Bill's Mashed Potatoes (chapter 9)

Day 13

▲ **Breakfast** *(Eat as much as you want.)*
—A banana and all the fresh fruit you want or fruit smooth-
ies or V8 juice and a couple of Wasa Light Crispbread or
Corn Thins with fat-free cheese melted on top.

● **Let's Do Lunch** *(Eat as much as you want.)*
—Soup of choice
—Salad of choice with dressing of choice
—Dad's Stuffed Peppers with condiments of choice
(chapter 9)
—Bill's Mashed Potatoes (chapter 9)

■ **Dinner** *(Eat as much as you want, but no protein entrée.)*
—A banana and fruit smoothies or fresh fruit
—Then, *if still hungry:* Patti's Refreshing Salad (chapter 9)

▼ **Evening snack,** *if still hungry*
—Frozen, seedless grapes and raisins or fresh fruit

Day 14

▲ *Breakfast (Eat as much as you want.)*
—A banana and all the fresh fruit you want or fruit smoothies. Try adding no-fat cottage cheese with your strawberries or other fresh fruit. Sweeten with Stevia. If fruit doesn't do it for you, try V8 juice with no-fat cottage cheese. Or try a little fat-free yogurt.

● *Let's Do Lunch (Eat as much as you want.)*
—Salad of choice with a few blue cheese crumbles and dressing of choice
—Veggies of choice
—Mom's Chicken Chow Mein with soy sauce (chapter 9)

■ *Dinner (Eat as much as you want,* but no protein entrée.)
—A banana and fruit smoothies or fresh fruit
—Then, *if still hungry:* Jim and Saunie's Antipasto (chapter 9)

▼ *Evening snack, if still hungry*
—Sugar-free Jell-O with assorted fresh fruit in it, topped with a little Cool Whip Lite

8

Stocking Your Shelves

Using the Ultimate Grocery Shopping List

W hat you don't have handy, you won't be likely to cook or consume when a craving strikes. That's a very basic principle of the *Let's Do Lunch* program. What you purchase and stock in your kitchen cupboards and pantry is very important. Keep only acceptable foods available.

Rather than focus on what you can't have, focus on what you *can* have. The list below includes dozens of foods, which can be combined into literally hundreds of dishes.

My wife is a reluctant grocery shopper. If she had her way, there would be no grocery stores—only restaurants and caterers. Below, however, is the Ultimate Grocery Shopping List so you can stock your kitchen and pantry shelves with foods for the *Let's Do Lunch* program. First, a few suggestions about purchasing various items:

Choose to Conquer the Store, Rather Than Be Tempted by It

When you go to the grocery store, go with your stomach full—preferably within an hour of eating. You'll be less prone to temptation. If at all possible, send another member of your family to do the shopping. That's the best way to avoid all temptation!

Shop the perimeter of the grocery store first. That's where you will find the fresh fruits and vegetables, meat, and dairy items. If given an option among fresh, frozen, and canned—go with fresh. You'll take in less sodium and preservatives and get a lot more taste for your dollar. When food tastes good, you don't feel as if you are depriving yourself.

After shopping the perimeter of the store, head for the frozen fruits and vegetables section. But try to steer clear of the frozen, prepared foods, including desserts, ethnic foods, and prepackaged dinners.

Shop the remaining nonfrozen-food aisles last. Head for the canned fruit and vegetable aisles. Avoid the aisles with cereals and packaged foods.

Tips for Purchasing Meats

When buying hamburger, also purchase ground skinless turkey breast. When mixed, the turkey takes on the flavor of hamburger, but you get a lot less fat in the recipe. I have found that ground meat tastes much richer if I:

- Buy sirloin steaks and ask the butcher to cut off the fat and put them through the grinder.
- Buy whole, boneless, skinless turkey breasts, and ask the butcher to put them through the grinder.

When Purchasing Items from Grocery Store Shelves

First, let me assure you that the names of foods in this section were specially selected by me, and they reflect my personal choice. Through the years, I have found these items to be the tastiest and healthiest foods for inclusion in the *Let's Do Lunch* program. None of the brands, menus, or restaurants have been paid a promotional consideration to be included in the program, nor does their inclusion in the program constitute an endorsement by them of this plan.

Second, I have discovered in talking to people from across the nation that many people these days have food allergies of some type. Do *not* include foods to which you have a known allergy.

The Ultimate Grocery Shopping List

Fresh Vegetables and Herbs
Alfalfa sprouts
Artichokes
Asparagus
Beets
Broccoli
Brussels sprouts
Cabbage of all types—both green and purple
Carrots—regular and baby
Cauliflower
Celery
Cilantro
Cole slaw in packages—preshredded, no dressing
Corn—frozen kernels or whole corn on the cob in packages
Cucumber
Edamame (soybeans with pods)
Garlic—whole bulb or "canned" minced
> *Note: You can find minced garlic in jars in most grocery store produce sections.*
Ginger root
Greens (collard, turnip)

Green beans
Jalapeño chili peppers
Jicama
Lettuce—Iceberg, Bib, Romaine; other leafy greens
Lettuce—mixed, in bag or loose (especially Spring Mix)
Mushrooms
Onions—green, white, yellow, red, or Vidalia sweet
  Note: No French fried onion!
Parsley
Peas—fresh, frozen, "snow"
Peppers—green, yellow, red
Radishes
Scallions
Shallots
Soy nuts (dry-roasted soybeans)
Spinach
Squash—spaghetti, summer, zucchini
Tomatoes—cherry, regular, grape size, sun dried (*no* oil)
Turnips
Watercress

What Not to Buy

No potato products—period. That includes potato chips, candied potatoes, hash browns, au gratin potatoes, French fries, mashed potatoes, scalloped potatoes, potato salad, potato tots, potato pancakes, and potato puffs. I didn't eat baked potatoes as I was losing weight. If you just have to have a potato occasionally, eat it with salsa, olive oil spray, I Can't Believe It's Not Butter Spray, or Butter Buds.

Fresh Fruits

Apples
Avocadoes

Bananas
Berries—blackberries, blueberries, raspberries, strawberries
Cantaloupe
Cherries
Grapes
>   *Note: Put some seedless grapes in your freezer.*

Grapefruit
Honeydew melons
Kiwifruit
Lemons
Limes
Mangos
Oranges—fresh and juice
>   *Note: Freshly squeezed juice is best.*

Papaya
Peaches
Pears
Pineapple
Plums
Raisins
>   *Note: Raisins are actually dried grapes, of course. You'll find,*
>   *however, that it's much easier to eat twenty raisins than*
>   *twenty grapes—in other words, it's easy to overeat raisins*
>   *without thinking twice about what you're popping into your*
>   *mouth. Eat raisins sparingly, and if given a choice, choose*
>   *fresh grapes.*

Tangelos
Tangerines
Watermelon

Canned and Bottled Juices
Apple juice (Dole)
Pineapple juice (Dole)

Tomato juice (Campbell's)

Vegetable juice (V8 100 percent and V8 Picante)

Note: If you like to create your own juices with a juicing machine—from either fresh vegetables or fresh fruits—you may also do so. Some grocery and health-food stores sell vegetable juices and fresh fruit juices. Just make sure no sugars have been added.

Canned Fruits

Applesauce—natural (Mott's)

Cranberry sauce—whole berry (Ocean Spray)

Fruits canned in their own juices or with light syrup—drain well before eating (Del Monte No Sugar Added)

Fruit cocktail—"lite," well drained (Del Monte Snack Size)

Mandarin oranges—drained and rinsed before use (Geisha)

Mixed fruit—in its own juice (Del Monte Chunky)

Frozen Fruit and Vegetable Products

Artichoke hearts

Blueberries (Big Valley)

Broccoli (Green Giant)

Cauliflower (Green Giant)

Cherries—dark, sweet (Big Valley)

Corn (Green Giant)

Edamame soybeans with pods (Sushi Bar)

Green peas (Green Giant)

Lima beans—baby (Green Giant)

Limeade (Minute Maid)

Mango juice (Minute Maid)

Orange juice (Minute Maid)

Raspberries—red (Big Valley)

Strawberries (Big Valley)

Sweet peas—baby (Green Giant)

Note: Do not buy sweet peas in butter sauce or cheese sauce.
Do not buy creamed peas.
Vegetables—mixed (Green Giant)

What Not to Buy

Do not buy sweetened fruits. Do not buy fruits canned or frozen in heavy syrup. Do not use bottled or canned cherries. Do not buy frozen vegetables that have been prepared with butter sauce or cheese sauce. Do not buy frozen Chinese-style veggies or Italian-style veggies. Do not buy any frozen creamed vegetables.

Canned Vegetables and Other Canned Goods

Albacore tuna—packed in water (Bumble Bee Fancy)
Artichoke hearts (not marinated)
Beets—whole, pickled, all natural (Greenwood)
Corn (Green Giant)
Green chiles—chopped or whole (Old El Paso)
Mushrooms (Green Giant)
Olives—black, pitted (Lindsay)
Peas (Green Giant)
Pumpkin (Libby's canned)
Salmon—pink, red
Sauerkraut (Bush's)
Skim milk (evaporated)
Water chestnuts (La Choy)

Beans

Baked beans (Bush's Deluxe Fat-Free Vegetarian)
   Note: Do not buy baked beans with brown sugar and molasses,
   with pork or tomato sauce, or canned "homestyle."
Bean sprouts (La Choy)
Black beans (Progresso)

Chili beans (Bush's Best Chili Hot)
Garbanzo beans—also called "chick peas" (Old El Paso)
Great northern beans (Bush's)
Green beans (Green Giant)
Kidney beans (Bush's)
Large butter beans (Bush's)
Lima beans (Del Monte)
Navy beans (Bush's)
Pinto beans (Bush's)
Refried beans—vegetarian or fat free (Old El Paso)
Three-bean salad—preferably without oil
> Note: If the three-bean salad is made with oil, then simply drain the oil off as much as possible.

Wax beans—cut (Del Monte)

Soups
Broth—beef or chicken (Campbell's or Swanson 99% fat free)
Chicken vegetable soup (Campbell's Home Cookin')
Lentil soup
Tomato soup (Campbell's)
> Note: Delicious when made with skim milk.

Vegetable soup—vegetarian or regular (Campbell's or Campbell's Home Cookin')
Note: I also eat Progresso Healthy Classics soups.

Tomatoes and Tomato Products
Chunky tomatoes—salsa style (Del Monte)
Stewed tomatoes—original recipe (Del Monte)
Stewed tomatoes—Italian recipe (Del Monte)
Tomato paste (Hunt's)
Tomato sauce (Hunt's)
Tomatoes—whole (Hunt's)
Spaghetti sauce—meatless (Healthy Choice)

What Not to Buy

Do not buy anything canned with fat, and do not buy any "combination" foods.

Seasonings

Basil—fresh, dried
Bay leaf
Blackened Redfish Magic
Blackened Steak Magic
Bouillon cubes—chicken and beef
Celery seed
Chili pepper (sometimes sold as red pepper flakes)
Chili powder
Cinnamon
Cloves
Cumin
Curry powder
Garlic powder
Ginger
Italian seasoning
Lemon pepper
Mrs. Dash seasoning
Mustard—Dijon, dry
Nutmeg
Onion—minced, powder
Oregano
Paprika
Pepper—black, white
Peppercorns—black
Poultry Magic
Pumpkin pie spice
Red pepper (also sold as cayenne pepper)
Salt—regular, sea, and seasoned salt (Lawry's)

Seasoning mixes—such as taco, chicken (Old El Paso)
Thyme
Vege-Sal

Salad Dressings, Sauces, Sprays, Spreads, and Condiments

All-fruit spreadable jams (Polaner)
Anchovy paste
Apricot puree spread (Polaner)
Barbecue sauce (Heinz or Hunt's)
Beano food enzyme drops

> *Note: This product will keep you from experiencing those embarrassing moments after eating something yummy that causes gas. You simply put a few drops on your first bite of the dreaded gas-causer, and eat to your heart's content, with no more worry of something leaving your body without your wanting it to. This product is available at health food stores and some drugstores. From now on you will be able to eat those wonderful gaseous foods that very seldom crossed your lips in the past!*

Butter substitutes (Butter Buds and I Can't Believe It's Not Butter spray)
Chili sauce
Cocktail sauce
Cole slaw dressing (Hidden Valley Ranch Fat-Free or Marzatti Lite Slaw Dressing)
Cornstarch (Argo)
Extract powder for baking and cooking
Fat-free salad dressings—French, Italian, Ranch (bottles or individual packets) (Kraft)
Fiber packets for beverages and foods

> *Note: A good source for these can be found on www.sweetleaf.com or call 1-800-899-9908.*

Fruit & veggie wash (Amway)

Honey
Horseradish
Hot peppers
Hot sauce (Tabasco)
Ketchup (Heinz or Hunt's)
Lemon juice from concentrate (Realemon)
Margarine—nonfat (Smart Squeeze)
Liquid Smoke
Mayonnaise—low fat (Hellmann's or Best Foods)
Mayonnaise dressing (Hellmann's Just 2 Good)
Miracle Whip Free Nonfat Dressing (Kraft)
Mustard—prepared yellow, Dijon (French's and Grey Poupon)
Newman's Own Salad Dressings
Oils—canola (Puritan), olive, safflower, Wesson vegetable oil
Olive oil cooking spray (Pam fat free)
Onion soup and recipe mix—dried, in packets (Campbell's)
Pickles—dill
Salsa (Tostito's and Newman's Own)
Soy sauce—lite (La Choy)
Spaghetti sauce, meatless
Steak sauce (A–1)
Stevia sweetener (in place of refined sugar)
> *Note: Stevia can be purchased at a health food store. It is 100 percent natural and is very sweet. Err on the side of adding too little rather than too much!*

Sweet relish
Taco sauce
Tartar sauce—low fat (Hellmann's or Best Foods)
> *Note: I like my own tartar sauce better. I make it with sweet relish and Kraft Miracle Whip free nonfat dressing. The recipe is in chapter 9.*

Teriyaki marinade and sauce (Kikkoman Lite)
Vinegars—apple cider, balsamic, seasoned rice (Nakano), red wine

Western Fat Free French Style Dressing
Worcestershire sauce: Lea and Perrin's

Bread, Cereals, Grains, Pasta, and Other Food Items

Cereals (whole-grain only)

Note: I did not eat cereals while I was trying to lose weight, but if you must have a little cereal occasionally, eat as little as possible and make sure it doesn't have sugar. If you need a sweet taste, sweeten the cereal with Stevia.

Crispbread (Wasa Light Rye Original Crispbread)

Note: If your grocer doesn't have Wasa, ask him to call 1-800-924-9272 and order it. I ate this fat-free bread with tuna salad, sometimes with chili and tomato soup, and at times my wife crumbled it up to use in meatloaf instead of bread crumbs. I didn't eat it with anything else because I believe that even fat-free pretzels, breads, pasta, potatoes, cereals, and other grains are fattening.

Dried beans with seasoning packets—assorted

Gum (Wrigley's Extra Sugarfree)

Egg noodles—yolk free

Note: Use these only if you are having a pasta or bread craving, and then as little as possible.

Popcorn (Orville Redenbacher's Gourmet Smart-Pop Microwave)

Real Foods Original Corn Thins

Rice—wild or brown (for very sparse use in making stuffed green peppers and cabbage rolls)

Rumford baking powder

Split peas—green or yellow

What Not to Buy

In general, I stayed away from breads, rolls, croissants, buns, muffins, biscuits, bagels, pasta, potatoes, noodles, crackers, cereals, rice, waffles, pancakes, and doughnuts. It is my firm belief that even fat-free breads, rolls, buns, muffins, bagels, pasta, potatoes, noodles, crackers, and cereals are fattening.

Meat and Poultry

Note: I stayed away from any meat that was not extra lean or at least lean—in other words, no meat with fat in it, no marbled meat, and no processed meat.

Beef
Filet mignon
Flank steak
Ground beef (extra lean)
Ground sirloin (ground sirloin steak after fat has been removed)
London broil steak
Porterhouse steak
Rump roast
Sirloin steak
Sirloin tip roast
Soup bones (with lean beef)
T-bone steak
Veal

Poultry
Chicken breast—whole or ground, without skin
Roasted chicken—no skin
Cornish game hen (no skin)
Lamb—lean
Turkey breast—whole or ground, without skin

What Not to Buy

I did not and do not eat pork or any pork-related products. In other words, no bacon, pepperoni, pork roasts, ham, or bologna.

The fat content in pork is very high, and many processed pork products are loaded with unhealthful nitrites.

Fresh or Frozen Fish

Note: I ate fish that was blackened, grilled, baked, or broiled— without any added fat.

Atlantic salmon
Brook trout
Cod fish
Flounder
Grouper
Haddock
Halibut
Orange roughy
Red snapper
Tilapia
Tuna—steaks or fillets
Walleye pike

What Not to Buy

I did not eat any fried or deep-fried fish. I also did not eat any fish that was baked or broiled with fat or that had been packed in oil. I avoided crab cakes, deviled crab, and scalloped oysters. In general, I avoided all shellfish because of my belief in what the Bible says.

Deli Items

Chicken—roasted or barbecued (skin removed)
Chicken breast—sliced, no skin (Healthy Choice)
Three-bean salad (drained before eating)
Turkey breast—sliced, no skin (Healthy Choice)

Beverages

Coffee—regular and instant, preferably decaffeinated

Soft drinks—*must* be sugar free (Canada Dry Diet Ginger Ale, Diet Rite Cola, which is sodium and caffeine free, Diet 7-up)

Tea—regular and herbal, preferably decaffeinated, *no* sugar added (Lipton, Celestial Seasonings [all types] and Diet Snapple iced tea)

> *Note: I have been told by nutritionists that diet, no-calorie green tea is the healthiest drink you can put into your system.*

Water—distilled, mineral, spring, and reverse osmosis "filtered" water

Wine—(Gallo Cabernet Sauvignon and Gallo Chablis Blanc, for use in recipes only)

> *Note: Distilled or reverse osmosis waters are the best. Plain old H_2O, bottled, or canned water without calories is next best. Tea is wonderful. Diet drinks are okay, but I stayed away from all other drinks with calories.*

Dairy and Eggs

American cheese (Borden fat-free)

Blue cheese—crumbled

Cheese as fat-free, processed food products (Borden Fat-free Sharp and Kraft Fat-Free Sharp)

Cottage cheese—nonfat or 1 percent fat

Creamers—nonfat (Carnation and Coffee-Mate)

Eggs

Egg substitute (Egg Beaters and Morningstar Farms Scramblers)

Gorgonzola cheese—crumbled

Milk—nonfat or skim

> *Note: Only use milk if you* must—*and then, as little as possible.*

Parmesan cheese (Kraft nonfat grated topping)

Sour cream—nonfat

Yogurt—nonfat (Dannon)
> *Note: Use yogurt very sparingly and only if you need a little with fruit, vegetables, or popcorn.*

What Not to Buy

Stay away from all other types of dairy products. I believe that even fat-free cheese is fattening, as are no-fat cottage cheese and fat-free yogurt.

Desserts

Cool Whip Lite
Gelatin—sugar-free (Jell-O)
Juice bars—no-sugar-added fruit juices (Welch's)
Popsicles—sugar free (Popsicle Ice Pops)
Yogurt—light frozen or fat-free frozen (Dannon and Edy's)

Vitamins

> *Note: Be sure to consult your physician or dietitian about your specific needs for nutritional supplements.*

Multivitamin and mineral tablet that includes vitamin D and iron
Calcium supplements (balanced with magnesium)

Simple and Delicious Recipes

Y ou are going to want to use *Let's Do Lunch* recipes over and over again! Most of these recipes are from family members and friends who have been on the *Let's Do Lunch* program. I've put in parenthesis specific products that I have used in making them. You may find other alternatives that you enjoy more.

Ultimately, you will want to experiment on your own and make up recipes so that you are eating "your way." I encourage you to do this. *Remember: choose the least-fattening foods that you enjoy eating.*

If you come up with a recipe of your own that you would like to share with the world, please send it to me (see page 184 for contact information). Please note: Any recipes you send cannot be returned, and you will not be compensated for them.

Also, you may keep up with new recipes and products by going to the Web site: www.letsdolunch.com. (Click on "message boards.")

Thanks and God bless.

Roger Troy Wilson

Recipe Index

Beef Recipes

Poultry Recipes

Fish Recipes

Egg Recipes

Vegetable Recipes

Dips and Sauces

Soup Recipes

Bobbi's Taco Soup

Ingredients:
1	lb. ground turkey breast (skinless)
1	onion
1	28 oz. can plain tomatoes
1	16 oz. can chili-flavored tomatoes
1	16 oz. can pinto beans, drained and rinsed
1	16 oz. can chili beans
1	16 oz. can corn, well drained
1	package taco seasoning
1	package dry Ranch dressing

Directions: Brown together the turkey and the onion—drain excess liquid. Add the canned vegetables and stir in the package of seasoning and the package of dry Ranch dressing. Simmer until flavors have blended. Serve hot.

Little Mary's Pizza Soup—A Must!

Ingredients:
1	tbsp. olive oil
1	medium yellow onion, chopped (1 cup)
2	small cloves garlic, crushed (or ½ tsp. garlic powder)
1	small green Bell Pepper, chopped (approx. 1 cup)
½	lb. lean ground sirloin or ground skinless turkey breast
1	cup sliced button mushrooms (fresh or canned)
¾	tsp. paprika
1	tbsp. dried basil

1 tbsp. dried oregano
½ tsp. salt
1 large (1 lb., 12 oz.) can diced tomatoes
1 large (1 lb., 13 oz.) can tomato sauce
½ cup sliced black olives, drained
1 can (14–16 oz.) pinto beans, undrained

Directions: 1. Heat the olive oil on medium/high in a large, deep saucepan with a lid. When it is melted, add the onion, garlic, peppers, turkey, and paprika. Sauté, stirring for 5 minutes until onion and meat are cooked. Add the mushrooms and cook for another minute.

2. Add the tomatoes, tomato sauce, salt & herbs. Cover and bring to a slow boil. While it is cooking, puree the pinto beans with a blender. Add this bean puree and 1½ cups of water to the pot. Simmer on medium-low for 10 to 15 minutes. Add the olives and gently stir in. If the soup is too thick for your liking, you can add another ½ cup of water.

3. Submerge a slice of Veggie Mozzarella cheese on top.

Little Mary's Chicken Corn Chowder

Unlike traditional chicken and corn chowder, this soup tastes fantastic without the fattening ingredients. It also contains a good quantity of beans (which you can't see or taste) and sweet kernels of corn, both of which will curb your cravings for bread, pasta, potatoes, and rice.

Ingredients:

2   cans (14–15.5 oz. each) cannellini beans, drained
1   cup Swanson fat-free or 99% fat-free chicken broth
1   yellow onion, sliced (approx. 1 cup)
2   cloves garlic, crushed or minced
3   tbsp. Willow Run Margarine or Smart Balance
1   large boneless, skinless chicken breast, diced into
      ½" cubes
1   cup fresh or frozen corn kernels
¼   tsp. ground bay leaves (or 3 whole bay leaves)
¼   cup low-fat or skim milk

Directions: 1. In a blender, completely blend together the beans and chicken broth until totally smooth. Set aside.

2. Melt the margarine in a large heavy saucepan. Add the onion and garlic, and cook over medium-high heat for 3 or 4 minutes. Add the uncooked, diced chicken. Sauté for 3 or 4 minutes more until all sides are lightly browned.

3. Add the bean/broth liquid, the corn, ground bay leaves, and a bit of pepper to the pot. Stir well and bring to a boil. Reduce heat to medium-low, add the milk, and simmer for at least 10 minutes more. It's done! (Remove bay leaves if you used whole ones.) As with all of my bean soup recipes, drink at least one or two glasses of water with or just after eating this chowder. It will make you feel really full and satisfied.

Eddie's Hearty Homemade Vegetable Soup

Ingredients:

2   small soup bones with lean meat
2   1 lb., 12 oz. can tomatoes (Hunt's)
1   cup sliced fresh carrots
1   cup sliced fresh celery
1   medium onion, chopped
1   16 oz. package mixed frozen vegetables—no
     potatoes (Green Giant)
4   cups water
2   beef bouillon cubes
5   peppercorns
1   bay leaf

Directions: In a large pot, combine soup bones, water, bouillon cubes, spices, tomatoes, carrots, celery, and onion. Cover and simmer for several hours until vegetables are tender. Remove bones and meat. Add package of mixed frozen vegetables—no potatoes—and simmer until they are tender. Refrigerate overnight and remove any fat that has come to the top before reheating to serve.

Great leftovers. This dish freezes well. —RTW

Little Mary's Cream of Mushroom Soup
(Deeelicious!)

Ingredients:

2	tbsp. olive oil
½	large yellow or sweet onion, finely diced
1–2	cloves of garlic, minced (optional)
1	8 oz. container of baby portabella or button mushrooms, sliced
2	cups boiling water
1	Knorr chicken or vegetable bouillon cube
½	cup white wine
1	cup 1% milk or low-fat milk
2	tbsp. corn starch
1	tbsp. fresh chopped parsley (or ½ tbsp. parsley flakes)

Directions: Heat the oil on medium-high in a large heavy saucepan. Add the onion and garlic. Cook for 5 minutes, stirring frequently. Stir in the mushrooms and parsley, and cook for 3 more minutes. Dissolve the bouillon cube in the boiling water and pour into the saucepan. Stir. Add the wine and milk, salt and pepper to taste as desired, and bring to a rolling boil for a few more minutes. Mix the corn starch with a few spoonfuls of water and pour into the soup. Boil for one more minute, and the soup is done. The soup only takes about 15 minutes from start to finish, which includes the preparation time. If you prefer a blended mushroom soup without the big pieces of mushrooms, you can use a hand-held blender at the end.

Little Mary's Thickest Tomato Soup
(Delicious, and you can't taste the beans!)

Ingredients:

2   tbsp. olive oil

1   large yellow onion, finely diced (1½ cups)

2   cloves garlic, crushed (omit if you don't like garlic)

1   large can (28 oz. / 794 g) crushed tomatoes

2   cans (14–15.5 oz. each) red beans, drained

¼   tsp. salt

¼   tsp. pepper

¼   cup loosely packed sliced fresh basil leaves or
    1 tsp. dried basil (optional ingredient)

Directions: 1. Heat olive oil on medium-high in large saucepan. Add onion and garlic, sauté for 3 or 4 minutes, stirring. Add crushed tomatoes, stir, and cover the saucepan.

2. Put beans in a blender with 2 cups of water. Blend until no pieces of beans are left. Pour into the saucepan. Add the salt and pepper. Bring to a boil, reduce heat to low, cover and simmer for 10 to 15 minutes.

If you want to add an extra depth of flavor, add the optional basil, stir in, and simmer for an additional 5 minutes. Yummy! —RTW

Joanie's Minestrone Soup

Ingredients:

1 medium onion, chopped

½ tsp. fresh minced garlic

½ tbsp. olive oil

1 can (14.5 oz.) ready-cut tomatoes (Hunt's)
   Note: You may use 2 cups chopped fresh tomatoes instead.

1 16 oz. package of frozen mixed vegetables—no potatoes (Italian style recommended)

2 cups tomato or V8 juice

1 cup reduced sodium chicken or beef broth (Campbell's)

1½ tsp. Stevia sweetener

1 tsp. Italian seasoning

1 tbsp. basil

⅛ tsp. pepper

1 15 oz. can navy beans (Great Northern), drained

Directions: In a large soup pot, sauté onion and garlic in olive oil over medium heat until onion is soft. Add tomatoes, vegetables, tomato juice, broth, sweetener, and seasonings. Bring to boil and add drained beans. Reduce heat and cover. Simmer approximately 20 minutes. If soup is too thick, add more tomato juice or water.

Make a large batch and freeze individual servings for use on days when you're on the go and have no time to cook. —RTW

Loerita's Quick Bean Soup

Ingredients:

1   16 oz. can Bush's pinto beans
1   16 oz. can Bush's great northern beans
1   14½ oz. can Del Monte stewed tomatoes
½   can water (7–8 ounces)
1   medium onion, chopped

Directions: Mix together. Heat to almost a boil, and then simmer approximately 30 to 45 minutes.

Suzie's Spicy Black Bean Soup

Ingredients:

½   cup chopped onions
1   green pepper, chopped
1   cup chopped celery
1   tbsp. olive oil
4   15 oz. cans black beans (Progresso)
1   cup chopped carrots
1   cup frozen corn
2   cloves garlic, chopped
1½   fresh tomatoes, chopped (*Note: You may use canned tomatoes that have been cut into smaller pieces.*)
4   beef bouillon cubes
½   tbsp cumin
½   tbsp. oregano

Directions: Sauté onions, pepper, and celery in olive oil. Add remaining ingredients. Mix and simmer approximately 60 minutes or until carrots are done.

Salad Recipes

Ange's Crunchy Waldorf Salad

Ingredients:
6   apples of choice, cubed
1   cup finely diced fresh celery
½   cup raisins (Sun-Maid)

Ingredients for Dressing:
⅓   cup low-fat mayonnaise (Hellmann's or Best Foods)
⅔   cup low-fat cottage cheese (1% fat or lower)
1   tbsp. lemon juice
1   tsp. Stevia sweetener

Directions: Blend together all the ingredients for the dressing. Then carefully blend the dressing with the apples, celery, and raisins. Chill thoroughly before serving.

Connie's Cobb Salad

Ingredients:

2	hard-boiled eggs, chopped
½	cup fresh green pepper, chopped
½	cup celery, chopped
1	large fresh tomato, chopped
1	cup frozen peas, thawed (Green Giant)
1½	cups diced skinless cooked chicken
1	medium-size head iceberg lettuce, thinly shredded
1	oz. finely crumbled blue cheese
	fat-free salad dressing of your choice

Directions: Hard boil and chop the eggs, and chop the vegetables. Dice the cooked chicken. Shred the lettuce into bite-size pieces and place in a large salad bowl or on a small platter. Arrange each of the vegetable, chicken, and cheese ingredients in strips across the bed of lettuce. Serve with your favorite fat-free dressing on the side.

Danita's Three-Bean Salad Delight

Ingredients:

1   15 oz. can wax beans, well drained (Del Monte)

1   15 oz. can green beans, well drained (Green Giant)

1   15.5 oz. can kidney beans, well drained (Bush's)

½   cup chopped red onion

½   cup chopped green pepper

½   tsp. white pepper

¼   tsp. Tabasco sauce

1   tbsp. Worcestershire sauce

1   cup fat-free Italian dressing (Kraft)

1   tsp. Stevia sweetener

Directions: Mix the three beans together with the onion and green pepper. Blend white pepper, sauces, and Italian dressing together, and pour over the bean mixture. Chill thoroughly before serving.

Diane's Chicken Salad with Grapes

Ingredients:

1½ cups cooked skinless, boneless chicken breast,
     chopped as finely as possible
1   cup celery, chopped as finely as possible
1   cup of grapes, each cut in half
½   cup fat-free or low-fat mayonnaise (Hellmann's Just
     2 Good)
     salt and pepper to taste

Directions: Mix all ingredients together. Chill well before serving. Serve on bed of lettuce or with Wasa Light Rye Crispbread.

Fred's Caesar Salad

Ingredients:

1   oz. egg substitute (Egg Beaters or Morningstar
     Farms Scramblers)
5   oz. olive oil
½   tbsp. minced garlic
¼   tsp. anchovy paste
½   tsp. red wine vinegar
½   tsp. lemon juice
½   tsp. black pepper
¼   cup fat-free Parmesan cheese (Kraft Nonfat Grated
     Topping)
½   tsp. Dijon mustard
1   head Romaine lettuce, shredded into bite-size
     pieces

Directions: Beat eggs on high speed. Slowly add olive oil while continuing to mix on high speed. Mix until smooth. Add all other ingredients one at a time until smooth. Add desired amount to shredded Romaine lettuce.

The dressing for this salad may be kept refrigerated in a covered container for 7 to 10 days. The dressing must be reblended each time it's used. —RTW

Joel Lynn's Seven-Layer Salad

Ingredients:
1   head lettuce, shredded
4   stalks of celery, finely chopped
1   green pepper, finely chopped
1   stalk green onion, finely chopped
1   lb. frozen green peas (Green Giant)
    (*Note: The green peas will thaw overnight in a salad.*)
1   cup low-fat mayonnaise (Hellmann's or Best Foods)
1   cup fat-free sour cream
1   tsp. Stevia sweetener

Directions: Layer the ingredients in a large glass bowl in the following order: lettuce, celery, pepper, onion, and peas. Mix the mayonnaise and sour cream together, and use this mix as the final layer. Sprinkle the sweetener over the top layer. Place in the refrigerator overnight for flavors to blend. Serve carefully from all layers.

Let's Do Lunch Fruit Salad

Possible Ingredients:
Apples
Blueberries
Cantaloupe
Cherries
Grapes, grapes, and more grapes
Grapefruit
Honeydew
Kiwi fruit*
Mango*
Oranges
Papaya*
Peaches*
Pears*
Pineapple
Plums*
Raspberries
Strawberries*
Tangerines
Watermelon*

Directions: Combine any, part, or all of your favorite fruit into a salad.

Some fruits are best combined with a fruit salad just before eating in order to keep them fresh and to keep the salad from becoming mushy. I've marked those salad ingredients with an asterisk (*) in the list of possible ingredients. Enjoy! —RTW

Mabel's Apple Tuna Salad

Ingredients:
1   6⅛ oz. can tuna packed in water (Bumble Bee)
1   small apple, finely chopped
3   tbsp. low-fat mayonnaise (Hellmann's or Best Foods)
    lettuce

Directions: Drain tuna and squeeze out all water. Separate tuna by rolling between hands. Add chopped apple and mayonnaise and mix together. Serve on bed of lettuce.
    I like this with sliced tomatoes on the side. —RTW

Martha's Broccoli Cauliflower Salad

Ingredients for Dressing:
2   cups (or less if desired) nonfat mayonnaise-style
    dressing (Kraft Miracle Whip Free)
5   tsp. Stevia sweetener
⅓   cup Kraft fat-free parmesan cheese
½   tsp. salt
½   tsp. basil leaves

Ingredients:
1   head lettuce
4   cups fresh broccoli florets
4   cups fresh cauliflower florets
1   bunch fresh green onions, chopped
1   can water chestnuts, drained and sliced

Directions: Mix together the ingredients for the dressing. Pour dressing over vegetables (except lettuce) and refrigerate overnight. When ready to serve, pour mixture over desired amount of cut lettuce.

Neet's Wild Rice Chicken Salad

Ingredients:
1   cup wild rice, uncooked, washed, and drained
5½ cups chicken broth
      juice of ½ lemon
1   boneless, skinless chicken breast, cooked, cooled,
      and cut up into bite-size pieces
4   green onions, sliced
½   red pepper, chopped
2   oz. snow peas, cut into 1-inch pieces

Ingredients for Dressing:
2   large garlic cloves
1   tbsp. Dijon mustard
¼   cup rice vinegar
¼   cup olive oil
½   tsp. salt
¼   tsp. Stevia sweetener
      freshly ground pepper

Directions: Cook rice in the chicken broth until done. While rice is cooking, blend together all of the ingredients for the dressing in a blender until smooth. Toss cooked rice with lemon juice. Add chicken, onions, red pepper, and snow peas to rice mixture. Toss mixture with dressing. Cover and refrigerate for 2 to 4 hours before serving.

Pat's Quick Coleslaw and Beans

Ingredients:
1   pkg. (approx. 16 oz.) coleslaw, washed
¼   small red onion, sliced
⅓   cup fat-free slaw dressing (Marzetti or Hidden
      Valley Ranch Cole Slaw Dressing)
1   16 oz. can pinto beans, drained (Bush's)
1   16 oz. can great northern beans, drained (Bush's)
1   15.5 oz. can kidney beans, drained (Bush's)
      celery seeds to taste

Directions: Mix coleslaw, onion, and dressing together. Add drained beans. Season with celery seeds or your favorite seasoning. Refrigerate several hours or overnight.

Patti's Refreshing Salad

Ingredients:
2   small heads bib lettuce (or lettuce of choice)
2   oranges
1   grapefruit
2   cups low-fat cottage cheese (1%)
1   tsp. Stevia sweetener

Directions: Wash lettuce and drain. In large bowl, tear lettuce into bite-size pieces. Peel oranges and grapefruit, and then tear oranges and grapefruit into bite-size pieces. Mix well. Drain fruit juices. Process cottage cheese and sweetener in a blender until smooth. Mix all ingredients together.

Shirley's Easy Fruit Salad

Ingredients:

2	20 oz. cans chunk pineapple in its own juice (Dole)
1	16 oz. can chunky mixed fruit in its own juice (Del Monte)
1	fresh cantaloupe, cut into bite-size pieces
1	fresh honeydew melon, cut into bite-size pieces
2–3	apples, cut into small, bite-size pieces
1	lb. seedless green grapes
1	lb. seedless red grapes
3	oranges, peeled and divided into individual sections
¼	cup raisins

Directions: Drain canned fruit and add to fresh fruit and raisins.

Tyra's Taco Salad

Ingredients:
½   lb. lean ground sirloin
½   lb. ground, skinless turkey breast
1   pkg. taco seasoning mix (Old El Paso)
1   can refried beans (Old El Paso), heated
2   cups or more chopped lettuce
½   cup chopped onion (optional)
2   small tomatoes, chopped
    salsa

Directions: Brown beef and turkey. Add seasoning mix and cook as package suggests. On a large plate, layer heated refried beans, then lettuce, cooked mixture, onions, and tomatoes. Top with salsa.

I use Danita's Salsa, of course—the recipe is with the Dips and Sauces recipes. You may also use ground white-meat chicken instead of turkey. It's great! —RTW

Beef Recipes

Brando's Lasagna

¼ lb. ground sirloin or lean beef

¾ lb. ground, skinless turkey breast (turkey will take on flavor of beef)

½ cup chopped onion

6 oz. can tomato paste (Hunt's)

2 5.5 oz. cans picante tomato juice (V8)

1 10¾ oz. can condensed tomato soup (Campbell's)

1 12 oz. low-fat cottage cheese (1% or lower)

2 tbsp. Parmesan cheese (Kraft Fat Free)

½ cup egg substitute (Morningstar Farms Scramblers)

2 tbsp. finely chopped fresh parsley

2 tbsp. finely chopped fresh basil

½ tsp. white pepper

5 medium zucchini, thinly sliced
Pam olive oil spray

1 12 oz. fat-free or skim, grated mozzarella cheese (Alpine Lace)

Directions: Cook the beef, turkey, and onion until tender. Add the tomato paste, tomato juice, and tomato soup to the mixture. Combine the cottage cheese, Parmesan cheese, egg substitute, parsley, basil, and white pepper, and mix lightly. Set aside. Place one half of the sliced zucchini in a layer in a 13" x 9" x 2" pan that has been sprayed with Pam olive oil spray. Follow with half of the cottage cheese mixture, half the mozzarella cheese, and half of the tomato/meat mixture. Continue with another layer, beginning with sliced zucchini and ending with the meat sauce. Bake at 350 degrees for 40 to 45 minutes.

Little Mary's Beef Potato Pie—A Must!

Ingredients:

½   lb. extra-lean ground sirloin

½   lb. lean ground turkey breast (skinless)

1   small onion, chopped (approx. 1 cup)

2   tbsp olive oil

2   ribs of celery, sliced

1   cup chopped, peeled carrots

2   cups fat-free beef broth (or 2 cups water & 1 Knorr beef bouillon cube)

1   tbsp. ketchup

1   tbsp. soy sauce

½   cup frozen peas

3   tbsp. corn starch

1   can (16 oz.) pinto beans, drained

2   cans (16 oz.) butter beans, drained

2   tbsp. Willow Run Soy Margarine or I Can't Believe It's Not Butter

Directions: In a large skillet, heat the olive oil on medium-high. Add the onions, celery, and carrots and sauté for 4 minutes. Add the meat and cook until browned. Drain off any fat.

Add the broth, ketchup, soy sauce, peas, and half of the pinto beans. Mash the remaining pinto beans with a fork and add to the skillet. Cover and simmer on low for 15 minutes.

Mix the corn starch in ½ cup of cool water. Add to the pot and bring to a boil. Stir until thickened (2 to 3 minutes). Add salt and pepper to taste. Remove from heat.

Pour into baking dishes (see following paragraph). Leave to cool while you make the topping and switch your oven onto 400.

Pour the butter beans into a microwaveable bowl. Add the Willow Run. Microwave on high for 1 to 2 minutes until the Willow Run is melted. Mash with a potato masher. Add a little fat-free chicken broth to make smooth. Spread the "LDL potatoes" over the top of individual deep pies or a 12" square Pyrex deep baking dish, around ½" to 1" thick. Put in the oven for 10 minutes to brown the topping.

Little Mary's Tamale Pie
(The topping tastes like mashed potatoes, and you can't taste the beans!)

Ingredients for the filling:
1½	tbsp. olive oil
1	small yellow onion, chopped
2	cloves garlic, minced
½	lb. lean ground sirloin
½	lb. ground skinless chicken breast
½	tbsp. cumin
¼	tsp. salt
½	tsp. pepper
1	tbsp. chili powder
1	can (14.5 oz.) crushed tomatoes
1	can (7 oz.) tomato sauce
1	can (4 oz.) chopped black olives
1	can (4 oz.) chopped green chilies

1   can (14 oz.) pinto beans, drained
1   cup corn

Ingredients for the topping:
1   cup corn
3   cans (15.5 oz.) large butter beans, drained
2   tsp. I Can't Believe It's Not Butter (Light)

Directions: 1. Preheat oven to 400 degrees. Heat the olive oil in a large pot on medium-high. Add the onion and garlic, and sauté (stirring) for 2 or 3 minutes. Add the meat, cumin, salt, and pepper, and cook for 5 or 6 more minutes until the meat is browned.

2. Pour pinto beans into a bowl. Mash them so they are kind of pasty with some whole pieces remaining. Put them in the pot along with rest of filling ingredients. Stir well, cover, and simmer for 5 to 10 more minutes.

3. Make topping. Melt the margarine. Put all of the topping ingredients, including the melted butter, into a deep bowl and beat with electric mixer or hand-held immersion blender. Blend until the beans are completely pureed (it's okay if some of the corn is left whole).

4. Uncover the filling and stir. Pour it into a deep Pyrex baking dish. Lightly spread the topping over the filling. Place in oven and cook (uncovered) for ·15 minutes. Remove from oven and let sit at room temperature for at least 10 minutes before serving.

Note: Omit anything you don't like.

Dayne's Main Dish Mexican Chili

Ingredients:

¾   lb. ground, skinless turkey breast (turkey will take on the flavor of beef)

¼   lb. ground sirloin or lean beef

½   cup chopped onions

2   14 oz. cans stewed tomatoes (Del Monte)

1   15 oz. can kidney beans (Bush's)

1   cup salsa (Tostitos or Newman's Own)

1   cup chopped celery

1   green pepper, chopped

1   tsp. chili pepper

½   tsp. salt

½   tsp. pepper

Directions: In a large pan, cook turkey, beef, and onions until the onions are golden brown and the meat is cooked thoroughly. Add the remaining ingredients. Simmer 20 to 30 minutes for flavors to blend.

Dray's Barbecue

Ingredients:

¾ lb. ground, skinless, white meat turkey (turkey takes on flavor of beef)
¼ lb. ground sirloin or lean ground beef
½ cup finely chopped green pepper
½ cup finely chopped onions
1 cup unsweetened pineapple juice (Dole)
1 tbsp. Dijon mustard
1 tbsp. Worcestershire sauce
1½ cups picante tomato juice (V8)
1 tbsp. cornstarch
¼ cup water

Directions: Cook the turkey and beef until browned. Add green pepper and onions, and sauté together with the meat. Once the vegetables are tender, add the pineapple juice, mustard, Worcestershire sauce, and tomato juice. In a small cup or bowl, mix the cornstarch in the water. Add the mixture to the meat mixture, and cook to thicken.

This mixture can be served as a lettuce wrap. To satisfy a bread craving, serve in half of a whole-wheat, rye, or whole-grain bun with the soft insides removed and discarded. —RTW

Jerry's Easy Beef Stew

Ingredients:

2   lb. very lean beef stew meat
1   28 oz. can tomatoes with juice (Hunt's)
2   medium onions, sliced
2   cups sliced fresh carrots
2   cups sliced fresh celery
1   6 oz. jar sliced mushrooms (Green Giant)
1   14.5 oz. can green beans (Green Giant)
3   tbsp. all-purpose flour
1   tsp. thyme
1   tbsp. salt
2   garlic cloves, minced
1   1.15 oz. package dry onion soup mix (Campbell's)
1   bay leaf
1   1-lb. package frozen peas (Green Giant)

Directions: Heat Dutch oven to 325 degrees. Cut stew meat into 1-inch cubes. Place meat, tomatoes, onions, carrots, celery, mushrooms, and beans into Dutch oven. Add flour, thyme, salt, garlic, onion soup mix, and bay leaf. Cover and bake for 4 hours or until meat is tender. When the mixture is thoroughly cooked, add package of frozen peas and heat until peas are cooked. Serve in a bowl as a soup or over a small amount of brown rice.

Neet's Meatloaf

Ingredients:

2	eggs
¼	tsp. pepper
2	tsp. salt
⅔	cup skim milk
3	slices Wasa Light Rye Crispbread, crumbled
1	medium onion, chopped
½	cup finely chopped carrots
1	cup chopped fresh portabella mushrooms
1	cup crumbled blue or Gorgonzola cheese
1	lb. ground turkey breast (skinless)
1	lb. lean ground sirloin

Ingredients for sauce:

2	tsp. Stevia sweetener
½	cup ketchup
1	tbsp prepared mustard

Directions: Beat eggs slightly. Add seasoning, milk, Wasa crumbs, onions, carrots, mushrooms, cheese, turkey, and beef. Preheat oven to 350 degrees. Form into one large round loaf on pie pan, or four individual oblong loaves in 9" x 13" pan. Bake 60 minutes for round loaf or 45 minutes for smaller oblong loaves. While meatloaf is baking, mix sauce ingredients. Spread sauce over meatloaf for the last 10 minutes of the baking time.

Roger Troy's Burgers

Ingredients:
½   lb. skinless turkey breast
½   lb. extra-lean ground sirloin
½   cup chopped onions
2   tbsp. barbecue sauce
⅓   cup crumbled Wasa Light Rye Original Crispbread
1   egg white
1   tbsp. mustard

Directions: Mix all ingredients thoroughly. Form burgers to desired thickness. Grill approximately 3 minutes on each side.

I eat these burgers without buns but with ketchup, sweet relish, tomato, and onion—and sometimes mustard. —RTW

Ron's Awesome Chili

Ingredients:
¾   lb. ground, skinless turkey breast
¼   lb. lean ground beef or sirloin
1   onion, chopped
1   cup chopped fresh celery
½   cup chopped fresh green pepper
1   16 oz. can kidney beans (Bush's)
1   15 oz. can chili hot beans (Bush's)
2   28 oz. cans whole tomatoes, cut up into smaller
     pieces
2   tbsp. chili powder
1   tsp. salt
1   bay leaf

Directions: Brown meat and onions. Add remaining ingredients. Simmer, covered, for three hours.
   This recipe makes great leftovers—and the dish freezes well. —RTW

R.M.'s Made Rights

(You have to try this one! You'll love it!)

Ingredients:

1   lb. ground sirloin or extra-lean ground beef
2   lb. ground, skinless turkey breast (turkey will take
    on the flavor of the beef)
1   medium onion, finely chopped
½   cup solidly packed, 100% natural pumpkin
2   10¾ oz. cans condensed tomato soup (Campbell's)
1   12 oz. jar chili sauce
1   tsp. pumpkin pie spice
1   tsp. pepper
1   tsp. salt

Directions: Brown beef and turkey. Add onions and cook until done. Drain off liquids. Add remaining ingredients and simmer for 60 minutes.

This recipe makes great leftovers. The mixture can be served as a filling for lettuce wraps. To satisfy a bread craving, serve in half of a whole-wheat, rye, or whole-grain bun with the soft insides removed and discarded.
—RTW

Sharon's Spaghetti

(Enjoy with or without meatballs.)

Ingredients for Sauce:

1   cup finely chopped onions
2   garlic cloves, pressed
1   tbsp. olive oil
1   28 oz. can whole tomatoes, chopped
1   15 oz. can tomato sauce
¼   tsp. black pepper
1   tsp. oregano leaves
1   tsp. salt (optional)
1   tsp. basil
1   tsp. herb seasoning
1   tsp. celery flakes
1   bay leaf
½   tsp. crushed red pepper

Ingredients for meatballs:

½   lb. lean ground sirloin
½   lb. ground, skinless turkey breast
½   cup crumbled Wasa Light Rye Crispbread
¼   cup skim milk
2   tbsp. finely chopped onion
1   tsp. salt
½   tsp. Worcestershire sauce
1   egg

Directions: In a large saucepan, sauté onions and garlic in oil until tender. Add tomatoes, tomato sauce, and spices. Simmer uncovered until sauce has thickened (30 to 50 minutes). Makes 4 cups. While sauce is cooking, mix ingredients for meatballs. Shape into twenty 1½-inch meatballs. Cook over medium heat, turning occasionally until brown, about 20 minutes. Then place the meatballs into a 400 degree oven for 20 to 25 minutes until light brown.

Rather than serve this sauce—or sauce with meatballs—over pasta, serve it over spaghetti squash. Place squash in oven (in a pan or on foil). Prick the squash with a fork to allow steam to escape as the squash bakes. Bake at 350 degrees until you can easily stick a fork into the squash (about 50 minutes). Then cut the squash in half and remove all the seeds. Scrape out the spaghetti-like interior of the squash with a fork. Delicious! —RTW

Steve O's Cabbage Rolls

Ingredients:

1	cup cooked brown rice (Success or Uncle Ben's)
½	lb. ground, skinless turkey breast
½	lb. ground lean sirloin
1	egg, beaten
¼	cup skim milk
¼	cup finely chopped onions
1	tsp. salt
1	large head of cabbage, washed

Sauce Ingredients:

1	16 oz. can tomato sauce
2	tbsp. Stevia sweetener
2	tbsp. lemon juice
2	tsp. Worcestershire sauce

Directions: Cook rice according to package directions. Mix together rice and all other ingredients except for the cabbage. Boil or steam the cabbage in a microwave oven for approximately 10 minutes or until a leaf can be removed easily. Then remove the core of the cabbage to make removal of leaves easier. While cabbage is cooking, mix together the ingredients for the sauce.

To form cabbage rolls, place a spoonful of the meat mixture into the center of a cabbage leaf, then roll up the cabbage leaf (similar to a burrito) or fold the leaves over the mixture to form small squares. Place the cabbage rolls seam-side down in a slow cooker. Pour sauce over the top of the cabbage rolls and cook on low for 7 to 9 hours.

Ty's Beef and Beans

Ingredients:
½   lb. lean ground sirloin
½   lb. ground, skinless turkey breast
1   cup chopped onions
2–3 16 oz. cans pinto beans (Bush's Best, drained well)

Directions: Brown beef and turkey. Add onions and cook until done. Drain off liquid. Add drained pinto beans and simmer for approximately 30 minutes. Season to taste.

Try this—you'll love it! I especially enjoy this topped with Danita's Salsa or with my favorite condiments. —RTW

Poultry Recipes

B.B.'s Chicken with Marmalade

Ingredients:
4   boneless, skinless, split chicken breasts
       no-stick olive oil cooking spray (Pam)
½   cup of orange all-fruit marmalade (Polaner)
½   cup fat-free Ranch dressing (Kraft)
½   package dried onion soup mix (Campbell's)
½   cup canned mandarin oranges, drained (Geisha)

Directions: Place chicken breasts in a 9" x 9" pan sprayed with olive oil. Bake for 20 minutes at 375 degrees. Drain off liquid. Blend the marmalade, Ranch dressing, and dried onion soup mix together in a blender. Pour over the chicken breasts. Bake at 375 degrees for another 20 to 30 minutes or until chicken is tender. Add the mandarin oranges during the last 5 minutes of cooking time.

This is one of my favorites! —RTW

Bob's Key Lime Chicken

Ingredients:
4   boneless, skinless, split chicken breasts
6   oz. can frozen lime juice (Minute Maid)
2   tbsp. honey
¼   cup unsweetened pineapple juice (Dole)
1   tbsp. Worcestershire sauce (Lea & Perrins)
1   tsp. lemon pepper
2   tbsp. cornstarch
4   pineapple slices

Directions: Place chicken in a shallow baking dish that has been sprayed with a no-stick spray. Bake at 375 degrees for 20 minutes and then drain off liquid. Blend the remaining ingredients (except pineapple slices) in a blender and pour over the chicken. Bake at 375 degrees for 25 minutes or until chicken is done. In the last 5 minutes of cooking time, add pineapple slices to chicken.

Edna Ruth's Chicken or Turkey
(This is made to taste like beef!)

Ingredients:
       skinless, boneless chicken breast (or turkey breast)
       Poultry Magic seasoning
1   10 oz. can Swanson's Lower Sodium Beef Broth

Directions: Rinse and pat dry the chicken or turkey breast. Sprinkle it lightly with Poultry Magic seasoning on both sides. Brown both sides in a pan sprayed with

Pam olive oil. Add a can of Swanson's Lower Sodium Beef Broth. Simmer the meat, turning it over several times, until both sides are fully cooked and tender. Shred the chicken or turkey. Again sprinkle it lightly with Poultry Magic seasoning and simmer 30 minutes more (adding more broth if needed).

This tastes so much like beef I almost put it in the Beef Recipes section! You won't believe how good this tastes—I eat it with a mixture of fat-free French dressing and my favorite mustard. —RTW

Ground-Chicken Sausages
(Taste better than fattening pork sausages.)

Ingredients:
8   oz. ground chicken breast (skinless)
½   cup drained and mashed pinto beans
1   egg (use Egg Beaters)
2   tsp. Morton's Sausage and Meatloaf Seasoning Mix
     (to order by phone: 630-595-8919)

Directions: Beat egg with fork. Mix in chicken, beans, and seasoning. Let set to thicken. Make into patties and fry on grill or pan sprayed with olive oil. Makes 4 patties.

Gayle's Chicken with Cranberries and Oranges

Sauce Ingredients:

1   11 oz. can mandarin oranges, drained (Geisha)
½   16 oz. can whole berry cranberry sauce (Ocean Spray)
1   4 oz. fat-free French style dressing (Western)
½   1.15 oz. pkg. dried onion soup (Campbell's)

Ingredients:

4   boneless, skinless, split chicken breasts
     Lawry's Seasoned Salt

Directions: Mix the sauce ingredients and refrigerate overnight. To cook the chicken: preheat oven to 350 degrees. Place chicken breasts in baking dish with lid. Cover and bake for 30 minutes. Remove from oven. Drain off excess liquid. Sprinkle chicken on one side with Lawry's Seasoned Salt, then smother chicken breasts in half of the sauce. Bake uncovered at 350 degrees for approximately 30 more minutes until chicken is thoroughly cooked and sauce is hot.

This is an excellent dish for entertaining—the sauce is made the day before.

The unused portion of the sauce may be frozen and used at a later time. You'll note that the sauce is made with only half a can of cranberry sauce and half a package of dried onion soup mix. I frequently double the sauce ingredients and then use only a quarter of the sauce in making the recipe. That leaves three more portions of sauce for later use! —RTW

Jack's Chicken Stir Fry

Ingredients:

4	boneless, skinless, split chicken breasts, cut into 1-inch chunks
½	cup white wine (Chablis Blanc-Gallo)
2	cups fresh snow peas
2	scallions, chopped
1	cup fresh carrots, sliced thin at an angle
2	cups fresh broccoli florets
¼	cup lite soy sauce (La Choy)
2	tbsp. shredded fresh ginger
¼	cup condensed chicken broth
½	8 oz. can water chestnuts, sliced
1	cup fresh mushrooms

Directions: Sauté chicken with the wine. Remove and set aside. Place remaining ingredients in a woklike pan and stir fry until just tender. Add chicken and heat until piping hot.

You won't need any rice with this stir-fry! It's hearty and crunchy and satisfying just the way it is. —RTW

Mary's Quick Apple Chicken

Ingredients:

4   boneless, skinless, split chicken breasts

2   tbsp. Butter Buds (liquid)

1   cup apple juice (Dole)

1   large onion, thinly sliced

1   garlic glove, minced

½   tsp. thyme

4   tsp. Dijon mustard

1   large apple, cored and thinly sliced

Directions: Flatten chicken breasts in a large nonstick skillet. Add Butter Buds. Brown the chicken. Add apple juice, onions, garlic, and thyme. Cover and cook for 10 to 12 minutes. Remove chicken from the pan and keep it warm. Bring the remaining liquid to a boil. Add mustard and apple slices; stir while mixture is boiling and until liquid is almost gone. Pour over chicken breasts.

Mom's Chicken Chow Mein

Ingredients:

4   boneless, skinless, split chicken breasts, cooked and cut into small pieces
1   10.5 oz. can condensed chicken broth (Campbell's)
2   cups water
1   chicken bouillon cube
2   cups coarsely chopped onions
3   cups coarsely chopped fresh celery
1   14 oz. can bean sprouts, well drained (La Choy)
1   5 oz. can sliced water chestnuts, well drained (La Choy)
1   lb. fresh or canned sliced mushrooms
2   tbsp. cornstarch
    brown rice (Success or Uncle Ben's)
    light soy sauce to taste

Directions: Sauté the chicken in a little chicken broth. Set aside. Put the rest of the broth, the water, and bouillon cube into a large pan. Add onions and celery and cook for approximately ten minutes until celery is tender. Add bean sprouts, water chestnuts, and mushrooms. Simmer, stirring frequently, for approximately 15 minutes. While mixture is simmering, cook rice according to package instructions. Add sautéed chicken to the vegetables and mix together. Add light soy sauce to suit your own taste. Serve chow mein over a small amount of brown rice.

If the sauce needs thickening, mix a little cornstarch with cold water and add it to the final mixture. This recipe makes great leftovers. —RTW

Ruth's Chicken Divan

Ingredients:
6   boneless, skinless, split chicken breasts, cut up
½   cup chopped onions
1   pound fresh mushrooms, cleaned and sliced
½   cup condensed chicken broth (Campbell's)
2   1 lb. packages frozen chopped broccoli (Green
      Giant), thawed and well drained
¼   cup low-fat mayonnaise (Hellmann's or Best Foods)
6   slices fat-free sharp cheese (Borden)

Ingredients for white sauce:
½   cup Butter Buds
3   tbsp. flour
1½   cups skim milk

Directions: Sauté the chicken, onion, and mushrooms in the chicken broth. Spray the bottom of a 9" x 13" pan with no-stick spray. Place the chicken/onion/mushroom mix and broccoli in the bottom of the pan. Mix the ingredients for the white sauce, then add the white sauce, along with the mayonnaise, on top of the meat and vegetables. Bake at 350 degrees for approximately 30 minutes. Add the cheese slices to the dish after it is cooked. Return to oven just long enough to melt the cheese. Remove breasts from pan with slotted spoon or spatula. (Whatever is not on top of chicken pieces when done baking, leave in pan and dispose. Don't eat the remaining sauce.)

Great leftovers! —RTW

Tyra's Chicken Parmesan

Ingredients:
4 boneless, skinless, split chicken breasts
½ cup skim milk
 Progresso Italian Style Bread Crumbs
 olive oil no-stick cooking spray (Pam)
1 15 oz. can tomato sauce (Hunt's)

Condiments to add according to taste:
 basil
 oregano
 salt and pepper
 nonfat Parmesan cheese

Directions: Preheat oven to 400 degrees. Dip each chicken breast in skim milk and then coat chicken breast in bread crumbs. Place in 10" x 7" glass pan sprayed with olive oil no-stick spray. Bake chicken for 25 minutes or until tender. Pour tomato sauce on chicken breasts. Season to taste with basil, oregano, salt, and pepper. Sprinkle with grated Parmesan topping in desired amount, and bake for an additional 5 minutes.

Fish Recipes

B-Bow's Bronze Fish

Ingredients:

1	cup low-fat mayonnaise (Hellmann's or Best Foods)
2	tbsp. lemon juice
1	tbsp. celery seeds
1½	lb. snapper fillets or any mild fish (such as flounder, grouper, or orange roughy)
	nonstick cooking spray (Pam)
½	cup nonfat Parmesan cheese (Kraft Grated Topping)

Directions: Preheat oven to 350 degrees. Mix mayonnaise, lemon juice, and celery seeds in small bowl. Wash fillets. Blot dry with paper towel. Arrange fillets in shallow baking dish sprayed with nonstick cooking spray. Spread mayonnaise mixture on each fillet. Bake for 15 to 30 minutes, depending on thickness of fillets, until fish is almost flaky when tested with fork. Remove fish. Sprinkle with Parmesan cheese. Return to oven for approximately 5 minutes. Then broil approximately 2 minutes to brown top. (Whatever is not on top of fish when done baking, leave in pan and dispose—do not eat.)

Charlie's Blackened Fish

Ingredients:

1	tsp.	chili pepper
1	tsp.	lemon pepper
¼	tsp.	curry powder
1	tsp.	salt
2	tsp.	paprika
2	tsp.	black pepper
1	tsp.	garlic powder
1	tsp.	onion powder
2	tsp.	red pepper
4	fillets of your favorite fish	

Directions: Shake all spices together in a large resealable plastic baggie. Add the fish fillets to the baggie and gently shake until each fillet is generously coated. Broil the fillets until the fish is just flaky. Serve with Hellmann's reduced-fat tartar sauce or Ty's Tartar Sauce.

David's Easy Grilled Halibut

Ingredients:

1	tbsp.	olive oil
2	tbsp.	lemon juice
1	clove garlic, finely minced	
1	tbsp.	fresh parsley
1	tsp.	black pepper
4	halibut fillets, approx. 6 oz. each	

Directions: In a large bowl, combine everything but the fish fillets. Place fillets on grill and then drizzle sauce over fish as you grill the fish. Cook approximately 4 to 6 minutes.

Del's Grilled Tuna

Ingredients:

4   tuna steaks, approx. 8 oz. each
1   tbsp. olive oil
      garlic powder

Directions: Preheat grill. Brush tuna steaks with olive oil. Sprinkle each tuna steak with garlic powder on each side. Grill approximately 3 to 5 minutes. Don't overcook—the tuna will be firm to touch and opaque. You may also blacken the tuna with your favorite Cajun or blackening spices.

Gordy's Baked Fish

Ingredients:

4   fillets of your favorite fish
½   cup green pepper, sliced into strips
½   cup chopped green onions
½   cup thinly sliced fresh carrots
1   lemon, thinly sliced
1   fresh tomato, chopped
2   tbsp. chopped parsley
½   cup chopped fresh mushrooms

Directions: Preheat oven to 350 degrees. Place fish fillets gently over two layers of aluminum foil on a very shallow pan or cookie sheet. Surround the fillets with the remaining ingredients. Bake for 30 to 40 minutes or until the fish is tender and flaky. Serve with tartar sauce.

Jim's Glazed Salmon

Ingredients:

2   tbsp. water
3   tbsp. concentrated orange juice (Minute Maid)
2   tbsp. lite soy sauce (La Choy)
1   tbsp. honey
2   tsp. olive oil
4   Atlantic salmon steaks, about 3/4-inch thick

Directions: Combine everything except salmon steaks in a small bowl to make dressing. Place salmon on ungreased rack or broiler pan. Brush with dressing. Broil or grill for 5 minutes. With large, wide spatula, turn salmon over carefully. Brush with balance of dressing and broil or grill 3 to 7 minutes or until fish flakes easily with fork.

Kitten's Tuna and Noodle Dish

Ingredients:
6   oz. yolk-free egg noodles (Mueller's)
½   16 oz. package frozen peas (Green Giant)
1   6 oz. can tuna packed in water (Bumble Bee)
½   cup sliced mushrooms (Green Giant)
2   slices fat-free sharp cheese (Borden)
1   tbsp. low-fat mayonnaise (Hellmann's or Best Foods)
       skim milk, as needed
       salt and pepper to taste

Directions: Prepare noodles and peas according to package instructions. Drain well. Drain tuna well and form chunks with a fork. Add tuna, cheese, mushrooms, and mayonnaise to hot peas and noodles. Mix together. (If the mixture is too dry, add a small amount of skim milk.) Heat thoroughly. Season with salt and pepper to taste.

Nancy's Tuna Roll

Ingredients:
3   hard-boiled eggs
1   cup packaged frozen peas
2   6 oz. cans white albacore tuna packed in water (Bumblebee)
5   tbsp. low-fat mayonnaise (Hellmann's, Best Foods, or Kraft Miracle Whip)
6–8 large lettuce leaves

Directions: Hard boil the eggs and thaw peas. Drain tuna thoroughly. Mix tuna, peas, and eggs with mayonnaise. Roll into lettuce leaves to make individual servings.

Tom's Ranch-Style Red Snapper

Ingredients:

4   snapper fillets
½   cup reduced-calorie French salad dressing
⅛   cup freshly squeezed orange juice
½   tsp. paprika
¼   tsp. ginger
¼   tsp. nutmeg
2   tbsp. fresh orange rind
    freshly ground black pepper

Directions: Spray a shallow baking dish with nonstick vegetable spray. Line with the fillets that have been carefully washed and patted dry. Combine the dressing, orange juice, paprika, ginger, and nutmeg in a blender. Mix for 30 seconds. Pour over the fish. Sprinkle with the orange rind and black pepper. Bake at 350 degrees for approximately 30 minutes or until fish is flaky.

Egg Recipes

Danielle's Deviled Eggs

Ingredients:
6   hard-boiled eggs
2½ tbsp. Marzetti Lite Slaw Dressing
½   tsp. dill
½   tsp. salt

Directions: Cut peeled hard-boiled eggs lengthwise into halves. Slip out the yolks and mash them with mixer. Add dressing and seasoning. Mix until smooth. Refill egg white halves with yolk mixture.
   Danielle says using a mixer makes the filling "fluffier."
—RTW

Decca's Delicious Eggs

Ingredients:
6   hard-boiled eggs
½   tsp. salt
½   tsp. dry mustard
½   tsp. paprika
2½ tbsp. reduced-fat mayonnaise (Hellmann's)

Directions: Cut peeled hard-boiled eggs lengthwise into halves. Slip out the yolks and mash them with seasoning and mayonnaise. Mix until smooth. Refill egg white halves with yolk mixture.

Popcorn-flour Pancakes
(Fluffy and delicious!)

In large bowl:
2   eggs (use Egg Beaters and beat with whisk)
Add 1 tsp. Splenda
Add ½ cup no-fat skim milk
Add 1½ level tsp. baking powder
Stir until baking power dissolves and batter becomes frothy
Add 2 cups of popcorn flour (see instructions below)
Stir until batter drops into small lumps

Use small amount of olive oil on heated griddle. Drop 1/4 cup batter on griddle for each pancake. Serve with blended blueberries or strawberries that have been sweetened with Splenda.

To Make Popcorn Flour:
Loosely place, 1 cup at a time, popped popcorn in Magic Bullet Blender (or power blender) until you have 2 cups of finely ground popcorn flour.

Vegetable Recipes

Bill's Bean Cakes with Salsa

Ingredients:

1½   tbsp. olive oil
1   small onion, finely chopped
¼   cup finely chopped red bell pepper
2   garlic cloves, minced or pressed
1   medium-size fresh jalapeño chili pepper, seeded
      and finely chopped
2   16 oz. cans pinto beans, drained and rinsed
¼   tsp. liquid smoke
¼   cup chopped fresh cilantro
½   tsp. ground cumin
¼   tsp. pepper
¼   cup yellow cornmeal
      olive oil cooking spray (as needed)
1   cup Danita's Salsa

Directions: Put ½ tablespoon oil in a nonstick frying pan over medium heat. Add onion, bell pepper, garlic, and chili pepper. Cook, stirring often, until onion is soft but not browned (about 5 minutes). Place beans in a large bowl and smash coarsely (smashed beans should stick together). Stir in onion mixture, then add liquid smoke, cilantro, cumin, and pepper. Mix well. Refrigerate until chilled.

Spread cornmeal on a sheet of wax paper. Divide bean mixture into 8 equal portions, and shape each into a cake, coating each cake with cornmeal. In the pan used to cook the onion, heat the remaining oil over medium-high heat. Add bean cakes and cook, turning until golden brown on both sides—approximately 10 minutes. If necessary, spray pan with olive oil to prevent sticking. Serve with Danita's Salsa.

Butter-bean Potato Cakes
(Taste better than potato cakes.)

Ingredients:
3   cans large butter beans, cooked and drained
1   cup frozen corn kernels, defrosted and drained well
⅓   cup finely chopped onion
⅓   cup finely diced green bell pepper
3–4 tbsp. of 99% fat-free chicken broth

Directions: Mash or blend the butter beans in a large bowl. (Tip: this is a great way to use up leftovers of the Bill's Mashed Potatoes.) Add the chicken broth and blend until they're smooth and creamy.

Add all of the other ingredients and stir together. Refrigerate the mixture for an hour before proceeding to the next step.

Make into patties, approx. ⅓ cup of each. This will make 11 or 12 patties.

Heat a skillet on medium-high with 2 tbsp. olive oil and cook patties on one side until browned. Turn over and cook on the other side until browned.

Jim and Saunie's Antipasto

Ingredients:
1   15 oz. can green beans (Green Giant), well drained
1   15 oz. can peas (Green Giant), well drained
2   tomatoes, chopped
¼   cup thinly sliced red onions
¼   cup sliced green peppers
    Nakano Seasoned Rice Vinegar (fat-free)

Directions: Mix first five ingredients together and then season with the rice vinegar. Let stand overnight in refrigerator.

Bills' Mashed Potatoes
(Taste better than mashed potatoes.)

Ingredients:
4   cans butter beans, cooked and drained
2   tbsp. Willow Run Soy Margarine or I Can't Believe It's Not Butter
2   tbsp. (or more) chicken broth
    dash of garlic powder
    dash of ground pepper

Directions: Put the butter beans and the Willow Run in the microwave until the Willow Run is melted. Mash with a potato masher or blend with an electric mixer, adding enough chicken broth to make creamy mashed potatoes. Add a dash of garlic powder and pepper and mix well.

Dips and Sauces Recipes

Danita's Salsa

Ingredients:
1	15 oz. can black beans, well drained
1	14.5 oz. can diced tomatoes, well drained
1	cup frozen corn
¼	cup seasoned rice vinegar
¼	cup chopped onion
1	4½ oz. can chopped green chilies, well drained
2	garlic cloves, minced
¼	cup sliced pitted olives (green or black), well drained
½	cup chopped jalapeños, well drained

Directions: Mix all the ingredients together and allow the flavors of the salsa to blend together for at least an hour before serving or eating.

I sometimes eat this salsa instead of a salad. This salsa is great over a can of drained and heated pinto beans. —RTW

Dorrie's Cocktail Sauce

Ingredients:
1	cup ketchup
3–5	tbsp. prepared horseradish
2	tsp. Worcestershire sauce (Lea & Perrin's)
1	tbsp. lemon juice

Directions: Mix well. Chill thoroughly.

For a little sharper taste to this sauce, you might add ¼ tsp. salt, 1 tbsp. lemon juice, and a few drops of Tabasco sauce (or more horseradish). —RTW

Mattie Lou's Curry Dip

Ingredients:

⅔   cup low-fat cottage cheese (1%)
⅔   cup low-fat mayonnaise (Hellmann's or Best Foods)
2   tbsp. ketchup
2   tbsp. honey
2   tbsp. grated onion
1   tsp. salt
7   drops Tabasco sauce
1   level tsp. curry powder

Directions: Mix all ingredients together in a blender and refrigerate overnight.

This is great as a dip for fresh vegetables! —RTW

Mike's Veggie Dip

Ingredients:
- ¾   cup low-fat cottage cheese (1%)
- 3   tbsp. low-fat mayonnaise (Hellmann's or Best Foods)
- 2   medium carrots, peeled and grated
- 3   small dill pickles, finely chopped
- 1   tbsp. caraway seeds
- ¼   tsp. pepper
- ½   tsp. salt-free Mrs. Dash, finely ground
       herbs and spices to taste
- 1   tsp. parsley flakes

Directions: In a blender, combine cottage cheese and mayonnaise and blend until smooth. Put remaining ingredients in a bowl—add cottage cheese and mayo mix. Do not process again in blender. Chill overnight. Serve with raw vegetables, especially broccoli, cauliflower, and carrots. Makes 1¼ cups.

Ty's Tartar Sauce

Ingredients:
- 1   cup low-fat mayonnaise (Hellmann's or Best Foods)
- ¼   cup to ½ cup sweet relish
- ½   tsp. grated onion (optional)

Directions: Blend together and refrigerate.
   You might try substituting Hellmann's Reduced Fat Tartar Sauce for this recipe. —RTW

About the Author

Roger Troy Wilson founded a multimillion dollar corporation, became a TV newscaster, a Club golf and tennis champion, and a partner in a Wall Street brokerage firm and an oil and gas company. He had achieved success after success in life, but just couldn't overcome his only meaningful failure . . . his obesity. Then, after trying and failing at diet after diet, he decided that because doctors and nutritionists hold such widely varying views on how and what to eat in order to lose weight, the only logical way to find the answers would be to use trial and error to discover what works and doesn't work.

With the help of God, he came up with those answers and wrote a book that reveals them—*Let's Do Lunch*. In the process, he lost 230 pounds and 24 inches from his waist and has kept it off for years. Wilson and his wife, Anita, reside in Bonita Springs, Florida.

To order more books or laminated recipe cards, to get an immediate personal response to questions, or to contact Roger Troy Wilson for speaking engagements or interviews, go to www.letsdolunch.com and click on "message boards," or call or write:

Sunshine Publications, Inc.
23924 Creek Branch Lane
Bonita Springs, FL 34135
(239) 390-3900
e-mail: roger@letsdolunch.com

You can also keep up with new recipes and new foods by going to the Web site.

If you go to www.letsdolunch.com and click on "message boards," you can read about and talk with other *Let's Do Lunch* dieters. Once you do, you'll want to get started on this program right away!